IMPOSSIBLE CHOICES

IMPOSSIBLE CHOICES

A Physician's Guidance on High-Risk Pregnancy in a World Without Roe

DAVID N. HACKNEY, MD, MS

The MIT Press
Cambridge, Massachusetts
London, England

The MIT Press
Massachusetts Institute of Technology
77 Massachusetts Avenue
Cambridge, MA 02139
mitpress.mit.edu

The MIT Press would like to thank the anonymous peer reviewers who provided comments on drafts of this book. The generous work of academic experts is essential for establishing the authority and quality of our publications. We acknowledge with gratitude the contributions of these otherwise uncredited readers.

This book was set in Adobe Garamond Pro by New Best-set Typesetters Ltd. Printed and bound in the United States of America.

Library of Congress Cataloging-in-Publication Data is available.

ISBN: 978-0-262-05470-6

10 9 8 7 6 5 4 3 2 1

EU Authorised Representative: Easy Access System Europe, Mustamäe tee 50, 10621 Tallinn, Estonia | Email: gpsr.requests@easproject.com

Contents

Author's Note

This book should not be construed as medical advice. One should not make real healthcare decisions based on nonreference texts, and descriptions from the past may no longer reflect modern management. Likewise, state and federal laws are continually evolving and would often change while writing this book, even from one draft to the next. Individuals in restrictive states should thus remain abreast of their current landscape rather than any specific information presented here. I have written the clinical cases in accordance with medical nonfiction practice, in which one avoids identifiable, specific patient encounters. My own story and those of public individuals are precise to my recollection or as reported in the media and court documents. Otherwise, vignettes are hypotheticals or composites by necessity, and they include aspects that are intentionally altered, simplified, or merged so as not to reflect real individuals. Such cases are still medically accurate and explore the genuine quandaries faced by my colleagues and by me. Finally, I am speaking only on behalf of myself, not any organization, and the views expressed are only my own.

An Intersection of Facts and Choices

I was standing in my kitchen in Cleveland on a Friday evening in June 2022 when the text messages poured in.

"How long until it goes into effect?" I asked a colleague.

"It's the law right now."

"Like, literally right now?"

"Yes, right now."

The United States Supreme Court had released the Dobbs decision that morning. The landmark ruling revoked the constitutional right to abortion, ushering in a new echelon of risk for patients and physicians. Soon after, Ohio's attorney general requested that the injunction previously blocking enforcement of Senate Bill 23 (SB 23) be lifted. The bill was a near-total abortion ban, with no exceptions for rape, incest, or fetal conditions, including life-limiting anomalies. SB 23 then became law that very same day, with no buffer zone or time for medical professionals to prepare—and I was on call that evening for maternal fetal medicine.

Colloquially referred to as *high-risk obstetrics*, maternal fetal medicine (MFM) is the subspecialty within obstetrics-gynecology (OB-GYN) that focuses on pregnancies with a wide array of complications. We see patients in preterm labor or with medical conditions like diabetes, lupus, cancer, and heart disease. We care for patients carrying triplets, or even higher-order multiples, and those who learn from screening tests that they are carrying a fetus with birth defects. I like to say that MFM addresses pregnancy plus any disease or complication existing under the sun. Because most of our days are spent ensuring that pregnancies successfully advance, issues related to abortion account for only a small percentage of my work. Likewise, only a small percentage of abortions occur in the context of fetal anomalies or maternal illness. However, there are a few million pregnant people at any time in the United States, thousands of whom are high risk, so my MFM colleagues and I still routinely confront questions and difficult decisions about abortion.

Medicine, at its most fundamental, lies at the intersection of facts and choices. When you describe the details of someone's disease you also describe, almost simultaneously, their choices now lying ahead. And there are always decisions to make, no matter how dire or absolute the reality—decisions ultimately made by patients rather than physicians.

For instance, in MFM, we often see people not yet pregnant but considering conception, but with a medical condition that could make pregnancy dangerous. For these patients, we will review their risks and likely obstetric management. We describe the impact of pregnancy on their own health and chances of an uncomplicated live birth. At the end of the visit, do we make a recommendation? Normally in medicine, physicians make recommendations after weighing the alternative clinical options. For example, my wife is also a physician, a practicing pediatric oncologist. When cancer strikes a child, she helps parents balance the risks of surgery against the risks of radiation, or chemotherapy A versus chemotherapy B, optimally in concert with clinical research and randomized trials. But for the MFM patient considering pregnancy despite risk factors, the two options are not equivalent to selecting between medications, or surgery versus radiation. It is the risk of pregnancy balanced against having or not having a child. Whereas my wife often makes a clear recommendation, I cannot equivalently counsel someone about their desire for children, as that is a personal choice transcending medicine itself. Some patients would reasonably never want children, making any risks from pregnancy illogical. Some, however, are willing to risk their entire health itself. In both cases, it is the patient's choice, not mine.

Likewise, when I diagnose a fetal anomaly and the patient is considering abortion, I provide as much medical information as I can, often requesting that pediatricians provide their guidance as well. What is the anticipated quality of life? How probable is survival? Would a child suffer? Beyond the medical facts, patients consider their religious beliefs, their support structure, and the impact that a medically complicated child would have on their family. I provide the professional information that I can—though ultimately, the patient needs to make a choice.

In that spirit, my goal in this book is to provide information so that the reader can make choices. The subject of abortion has bountiful viewpoints, intersects lives in numerous ways, and is approached from many different fields of study. For example, there are patient stories; the labors of lawyers and activists; and many important cultural, economic, gender, and societal perspectives. Even within medicine, there are my colleagues in gynecology who face legislation's impacts on contraception, infertility specialists concerned about in vitro fertilization, and physicians who dedicate themselves to abortion care for all patients. This book is about my field of maternal fetal medicine, written by a high-risk obstetrician about pregnancy complications—both broadly and in the critical ways in which they are impacted by abortion bans after the Dobbs decision. High-risk obstetrics impacts everyone. Any healthy pregnancy, for example, can become high risk at any moment as many complications arise randomly and unpredictably. Thus, the millions of pregnant or pregnancy-capable people living in states with abortion bans need to familiarize themselves with common complications in case one should occur or when weighing the initial decision to conceive. What if you or a pregnant loved one find themselves bleeding or with preeclampsia or a congenital fetal anomaly? What if you are pregnant with a preexisting medical condition or are suddenly exposed to a virus that can cross the placenta to damage the fetus? What are the risks, what are the laws, and what are the decisions that you and your doctors will then have to make?

Obstetrics is also importantly not siloed within medicine, and medicine is not siloed within a society. The criminalization of medicine should concern all physicians, and the diminution of freedoms should alarm all citizens. Even if a doctor is not an obstetrician, they likely still regularly see and manage pregnant patients, including in issues related to abortion. Since the Dobbs decision, oncologists have weighed the legal risks of abortion for patients with cancer and cardiologists for patients experiencing heart failure. Emergency medicine physicians are now the front line of legal battles surrounding pregnant patients walking into ERs. For patients who are not themselves capable of pregnancy or not living in states currently under bans, they and their healthcare also may not be immune to future expansions of legislative interference.

Before everything else, there was that first day in June 2022. Standing in my kitchen, I quickly had to think about the world after Roe into which we had been thrown. Inevitably, I did later have my first patient who was pregnant, previable, and had a life-threatening complication under this new ban. I remember standing outside her door, gathering my thoughts before walking in. I was going to have to make medical choices balanced against legal jeopardy. Whatever the future was going to be after Roe was here now.

I BEFORE AND AFTER DOBBS

1 RISK: WHAT MAKES A PREGNANCY "HIGH RISK"?

Maternal fetal medicine specialists, also known as high-risk obstetricians, manage pregnancies with a wide range of complications. Compared to practitioners of medicine as a whole, there are not many of us in the United States: around three thousand physicians, as estimated from professional society membership,[1] with a little over one hundred new fellowship graduates each year. Our country would benefit from larger numbers as demographic and medical trends have made our obstetric population progressively higher risk. Likewise, the geographic density of high-risk physicians is associated with improved pregnancy outcomes, including maternal mortality.[2] However, the educational road leading to maternal fetal medicine is long. Each of our new graduates has had to complete, following college itself, four years of medical school, then four of OB-GYN residency, followed by three additional years of high-risk fellowship—all in all, over a decade of postbaccalaureate education.

What do high-risk obstetricians do upon finally graduating? They perform an array of fascinating activities, with one day always different than the next. On a Monday, I may be in the operating room performing surgery in sterile gown and scrubs, then on a Tuesday, in an outpatient office, managing pregnant patients with problems ranging from hypertension to diabetes to lupus. The next day may be a fetal ultrasound day, with me sitting quietly in a dark room drinking coffee while reviewing the sonographer's black-and-white images on large screens. The day after, I perhaps have no patient responsibilities at all, my hours focused on research, administration, or teaching medical students, residents, and fellows.

On days that I see patients in the office, who are the patients that I see? When would you or a loved one be seen by myself or one of my colleagues in MFM? It is not always straightforward. Sometimes this question is answered administratively, since within a healthcare system complications may formally trigger referral. Guidance on consultation also exists from the American Academy of Pediatrics and the American College of Obstetricians and Gynecologists.[3] Otherwise, different general obstetricians vary in the exact conditions they may or may not feel comfortable managing. For example, some will manage gestational diabetes themselves, and some will always refer. A good rule of thumb is that if a pregnant patient has risk factors or is simply worried about the course of care, it is always reasonable to ask if an MFM consultation is appropriate. Unfortunately, the answer may be influenced by geography. For patients in rural communities, the nearest high-risk obstetrician can be a prohibitive distance away. When I was a fellow in Pittsburgh during the mid-2000s, there were exceedingly few MFM specialists in the northern half of West Virginia, with patients driving hours over mountain roads to see us. After Dobbs, many states are also at risk of losing providers as they flee criminal jeopardy, tragically leaving behind vulnerable patients. For patients who do find themselves geographically isolated, telemedicine options are becoming increasingly common.

What if instead one resides in a large city where local MFM practitioners are abundant and a pregnant patient could, themselves, decide if she was or was not "high risk?" "Am I high risk?" is among the questions I most often face. Perhaps the patient wants to know who to see for prenatal care or are unsure about continuing the pregnancy. Patients and the public often ask at which degree of risk a physician would consider recommending abortion.

Sometimes "high risk" is obvious—or, like the famous Supreme Court definition, you know it when you see it. Among the highest-risk patients I have cared for are a handful whose heart or lung disease was so severe that prior to pregnancy they had undergone tracheostomies. A plastic devise protruded from the bottom of their neck, the hole from which was covered by their hand when they wanted to talk. One night on call, I found myself running back and forth between labor and delivery and the intensive care unit (ICU). In the labor and delivery unit were mostly healthy patients experiencing term labor. In the ICU, by contrast, was a pregnant woman with severe lung disease, now intubated through the tracheostomy in her neck. She had made it far enough that we were inducing labor in an effort to deliver safely. Although people often presume cesarean delivery is preferable in critically ill patients, a successful vaginal delivery will often place less overall stress on the body. Thus, with the patient attached to the ventilator, we placed an epidural for pain relief and started contraction medications. If we could keep labor progressing normally while also helping her breathe with the machine, then we could get through this—but that night, it was not working. Her body was not handling labor, but at the same time I worried she could worsen under the strain of a cesarean if we operated instead. So, we kept adjusting the ventilator, continuing with labor, and then readjusting the machine settings when she worsened again, myself moving back and forth between labor and delivery and the ICU, riding the elevator up and down. While standing in labor and delivery, I got another call that she was worsening, her oxygen levels dropping. I started to ride the elevator back up to the ICU.

She is going to die, I thought to myself, leaning exhaustedly into the elevator's corner. *Should we try a cesarean instead? Should we further change the ventilator settings?* All options had terrible trade-offs. At that time, many years ago, I had not yet had a mother die while directly under my care, and I realized suddenly that I was not prepared for this. So in lieu of continuing to perseverate about labor and ventilator settings, I had to think about myself for that minute in the elevator.

Medical practice can be a series of tragic experiences to which you adjust over time. You experience something terrible, then develop a strategy, and then hope to cope better the next time. I had not been here before, however; I needed a framework. But what is the framework through which we view risk?

What if one day, instead of someone with a tracheostomy or similar severe condition, a completely healthy pregnant patient has been scheduled in my office by mistake? What would her risks be? This patient takes no medications other than vitamins, has no symptoms, no concerning family history, and holds in her hand reassuring laboratory and radiology results. What risks does pregnancy impose upon her?

One the most common and serious complications, preeclampsia, occurs 7 to 8 percent of the time, though often in patients with specific risk factors such as diabetes or hypertension. However, in one study, the risk of preeclampsia was still 4.4 percent, almost one in twenty, among patients for whom not a single risk factor could be identified.[4] In another large study of completely healthy patients, 0.2 percent still had bleeding at delivery sufficient to require a blood transfusion, and 0.1 percent had complications requiring admission to an ICU.[5] Although it is even more uncommon, completely healthy pregnant patients will still sometimes die.

So, if that hypothetical healthy patient asks me if they could develop a blood clot, or preeclampsia, or sepsis, or even die, the answer is never technically no. This, in part, is why it is so critical to extend reproductive freedoms to all individuals, not just those at high risk, as all pregnant patients face risk. However, if the scale of risk never reaches zero, then where does my subspecialty draw a line between the patients we do and do not see?

Some professions date back hundreds if not thousands of years. In Western traditions, medicine as a whole classically begins with the school founded by Hippocrates in Kos over two thousand years ago. My specific field of high-risk obstetrics, by contrast, is only as old as I am: I myself was born in 1973, the same year the American Board of Obstetrics and Gynecology formalized plans for certification in maternal fetal medicine. As a medical student surveying the array of specialties from which to choose, it is easy to forget that they are all fundamentally human inventions. The field of cardiology didn't just arise organically from the earth; rather, medicine drew an imaginary circle around the heart then selected for the name the Greek over the Latin root. Almost all medical specialties are defined by an organ system or patient demographic. The gerontologist cares for the elderly, the pediatrician the young. Demarcations based upon some degree of risk, however, are less straightforward. My wife, for example, cares for children with cancer. If a pathologist sees under their microscope a cancer cell found in someone under eighteen years of age, then that child is now her patient. But in MFM, we must instead draw our circles using risk. So fundamentally, then, what is risk?

When I was a fellow and master's student at the University of Pittsburgh, I was both training clinically in maternal fetal medicine and taking statistics classes at the same time. During the day, I would do the rounds of the "high-risk" pregnant patients admitted to the hospital's "high-risk" unit; then in the lecture hall, I would learn from a statistician what risk actually was.

Risk is the marriage between what we know and what we do not. To perceive risk requires at least some knowledge: the facts that floors are slippery, cars may crash, patients acquire disease. Simultaneously, you do not know the outcomes, the confounders, the future; risk exists in exactly that intersection between known and unknown. And uncertainty is often multilayered, more convoluted than just not yet knowing what may happen.

As an example, imagine you are about to roll a die in your hand. There exists no knowledge of what the number will be, and thus you face uncertainty—but looking at the die, you understand the probabilities you face. Now imagine that held in your hand is either a die or a coin, but with your hand closed, you cannot tell which. Now you face two layers of uncertainty: uncertainty of the outcome, but also, more fundamentally, uncertainty of the underlying probabilities themselves. Are your chances one in six or one in two? In Dungeons and Dragons, players famously employ an array of unusual dice, ranging from a pyramid to a twenty-sided die resembling a small ball. What if you held some dice in your hand, but now had no idea what they were at all?

As medical technology advances, more patients are now living with conditions that were previously lethal. In my career, I have seen patients among the first to enter adulthood with rare pediatric diseases, which children have only recently survived under modern therapies. Their condition is still present but controlled sufficiently that they venture first into adolescence, then tentatively early adulthood, then even later into my office considering pregnancy. However, no similar prior pregnancies have ever been reported on account of their disease being uncommon and previously fatal. So, if such a patient is considering abortion, how do I counsel that patient on obstetric risks? How does that patient rationally make a decision? I study their disease to my best ability and draw plausible assumptions from physiology or related illnesses, but ultimately it is a best guess; neither the patient nor I know which dice are held in our hands.

The risks of medications in pregnancy are also often unknown. Hypothetically, what if scientists develop a wonderful new medication tomorrow that allows patients to experience enhanced control of their disease, but it has no obstetric data when first released as pregnant patients were excluded from early trials? How long from this starting point will it take to accumulate pharmacologic data on pregnancy? Years? Decades, even? To start, you need the initial pregnant patients using the medication, usually due to a combination of the result of inadvertent circumstances and patients who cannot safely discontinue. When those first patients deliver, you will then have some obstetric data but still no information on childhood or pediatric outcomes. If you want to know the risks of a medication's pregnancy exposure on children five or ten years of age, you have no choice but to wait five or ten years. This is a common, nonhypothetical problem faced in MFM, with innovations thankfully bringing new medications to market, but always years away from obstetric data. Thus, we and our patients often must make medication decisions with uncertainty.

However, both mathematically and in life, risk is meaningless without time. For a statistician there never just exists "risk" as an abstract, floating number independent of the elapse of time; instead, risks are always defined relative to some beginning and end. The risk of driving to the hospital persists only until you exit your car. Risks of pregnancy exist for the duration of pregnancy. In one *Twilight Zone* episode, the protagonist has a stopwatch that, when clicked, freezes time for everything other than himself; it is used subsequently in the story for mischief and theft. If held in our own hands, all our risks would simply vanish when we click the stopwatch, risk becoming inconsequential absent the passage of time. If facing a decision, we could just sit and ponder, or wander through libraries full of books.

The interdependence of risk and time is felt strongly in obstetrics where decisions are always made with the pregnancy continually advancing. If someone wants to consult the city's best orthopedic surgeon for their shoulder, they may face a six month wait for that coveted first appointment. In obstetrics, the whole pregnancy might conclude in the same time frame. Thus, when pregnant patients are referred to high-risk specialists, we do our logistical best to see them quickly; likewise, when our patients require other specialists, we often pull strings to expedite the process. We always hear the ticking clock.

Opponents of abortion likewise long ago recognized the value of weaponizing time. Many states have twenty-four-hour waiting periods that serve no necessity; there are telemedicine bans that force patients to spend time traveling; and victims of rape or incest are required to spend time filing formal police reports. Even in many states that are otherwise permissive, places where abortion remained legal after Dobbs, pointless and problematic twenty-four-hour waiting periods still existed. In theory these could prevent impulsive decisions that a person would later regret. However, no evidence for such benefit exists; abortion itself is not associated with high degrees of regret, and the vast predominance of patients are unequivocally certain when walking through the doors. This is especially true for those traveling great distances. As bans spread across the country after Dobbs, waiting periods in otherwise permissive states became formidable barriers, adding critical hurtles for patients already traveling, already having to make decisions against vanishing time.

Once, I was scheduled to see a patient considering pregnancy in the context of herself having an incurable disease; she was undecided about conceiving. Although her illness would inevitably progress and one day be fatal, some patients could still survive many years, if not even a few decades, given temporizing treatments and the disease's potential to remain stable for times. However, even when dormant, the disease was always present, always lurking somewhere, never to be vanquished. I reviewed her chart extensively the day before her visit. Currently, she was in good overall health: the disease for now at bay, her medications safe for use in pregnancy. Scrolling through her records, I found a survival prediction from the week prior. Essentially, her physician had entered into a computer a wide swath of variables: her age, her weight, how long she had already had the disease, results from recent laboratory testing, and so on. A statistical model then estimated the number of years she was likely to live. The resultant estimate was that she would survive another three to six years. Great, I thought: Everything right now looked perfect. She was currently stable, and if she conceived, she would likely have a healthy outcome—though she would need to decide soon as her future was uncertain. However, with a survival estimate of three to six years, she would still spend time with her child before passing away. In his moving memoir, *When Breath Becomes Air*, Dr. Paul Kalanithi, a neurosurgeon facing incurable lung cancer, decides with his wife to have a child despite the certainty of his prognosis. Later in the book, he espouses the joy of even the short time of his final days with his daughter, in the end happily imagining the life she would live beyond him. Thus, I found the concept of this patient and her husband electing to travel such a road touching, and I looked forward to the next day's visit.

In the office with her that morning, I reviewed her history, confirmed her medication list and absence of symptoms, and then discussed how a pregnancy would be managed in the context of her illness. I told her I did not see a contraindication to them conceiving at this time, with a pregnancy most likely resulting in a medically uneventful birth. She and her husband smiled nervously, though excitedly, holding hands, exchanging knowing glances. As the conversation was wrapping up, I alluded to hopefully seeing them back again soon. She said they were anticipatory, though, not actually planning to conceive yet for a year or two; they still wanted to enjoy some time themselves as newlyweds without children. I said that a year to two years could be more complicated and uncertain. She was confused, the happy conversation unraveling as we increasingly perceived a disconnect. Perhaps mistakenly, I made mention of the statistical survival estimate in her chart.

"What estimate are you talking about?" she said, no longer smiling at all.

She had not yet actually seen her newest model or lab results. Later I would learn she had a scheduled, upcoming appointment with her specialist, at which time he planned to break the news gently and in person rather than over the phone. Her disease was not my own area of expertise, let alone the survival statistics, so I attempted initially to dodge as I was not the most appropriate physician with whom to review the information. However, she now reasonably wanted to see her report. Sitting in my chair, looking at her estimates on my screen, I realized I could not justify preventing her from also seeing them if desired. I told her before rotating my monitor that this was only mathematical modeling—that these results can be wrong, that this was not my own specialty—then slid around the screen for her to read, her eyes starting at the top, scrolling to the bottom, and then to the final survival estimate of three to six years, followed by the signature of her physician. She did not cry that day, but her face lost all color and expression. She sat perfectly still. I realized I had misinterpreted everything. Her goal had not been for a child to warm her heart in just her final days, their imagined future with her husband encircling her in comfort as she passed away, a happy dream into which one slides. No, her goal had been to sit in bleachers during sporting events, attend high school graduation, maybe walk down an aisle, all now dissolving away along with time itself.

I told her that everything I said during the visit was still true, that now would be a reasonable time to conceive if she wanted a child, though if the estimate was accurate, it would be best to decide within the next year. This was many years ago. I do not remember how many, though more than three—and more than six. I never saw her again.

Maybe she did ultimately have a child through a different physician, maybe in a different city. Maybe the statistics were wrong, and she is still alive somewhere today. However, presuming she has passed away without children, I hope it was because she made the active decision to do so—that it was not an outcome of default as she remained conflicted, undecided, depressed, perhaps, as time ran out. A story in which someone young and in the prime of life is unfairly stuck down by disease is tragic, though not necessarily more so by having made the choice to not have children; stories that do not end with children are not automatically sad endings. I hope that if she did not conceive, it was because to do so was not consistent with her goals in the years she had left; that if she was facing limited time, she did not want to spend it pregnant, recovering from a delivery, being up through the night with breastfeeding and diapers. I would like to imagine instead long walks talking with her husband, brunch with old friends, reading the book she had always wanted to read, seeing the towns she had always wanted to visit.

In studying statistics, you learn to see the world as uncertain, never completely predictable, subject to influence from confounders measured and unmeasured. Statistics are at the same time intricate yet supremely humble, almost a philosophy or worldview more so than a precise mathematical proof. Algebra, trigonometry, and calculus certainly play roles in a universe filled with angles, triangles, and waves, but in our day-to-day lives we think constantly of our chances, outcomes, and probabilities. So much of medicine itself, let alone obstetrics or reproduction, hinges upon our risks. As a physician, I can quantify risk, and I can describe risk, but in the end, I cannot answer the question of how to live.

On that night with the laboring tracheostomy patient in intensive care, I contemplated her early pregnancy as I rode the elevator up to the unit. I had seen her back at the very beginning. I had counseled her about the grave risks of pregnancy with her heart and lung disease. I had told her she could potentially die during labor. Inevitably, she would need to deliver, vaginally or by cesarean, which would place a significant stress on her body. It was like telling someone with heart disease that several months from now they will be forced to run a marathon, and once they start running, they cannot stop until they cross the finish line. They would have to keep running even if they worsen, even if they stopped being able to breathe on their own. Thus, despite all our technology, and all our medications, sometimes patients do not survive. But I also told her everything could go well, that these outcomes were difficult to predict. She was at high risk, but risks themselves are not always certainties.

With all that information, she made the decision back then to continue. It was her choice to make and not mine. Now that we were here at the end, I had to respect that choice, even if it was not the decision I would have made myself. How many times had I supported patients who decided to not continue their pregnancies? How many times did I tell them they were choosing reasonably, that nobody should judge them for the decision they were making? If I supported those patients in the past, then I needed to support this patient now. And if she was going to die that night, then I needed to support her all the more.

As I walked into the room, she signaled that she needed to push. She was completely dilated and had an uncomplicated delivery a few minutes later. Over the next forty-eight hours, her ventilator settings improved. She left the hospital alive with her child. On a busy day in labor and delivery, you can deliver several babies in a single shift, day after day. But looking at the glowing faces of the other workers in the ICU that night, the nurses and physicians who see far more deaths than births, I realized how easy it is to forget what a momentous event this really is.

2 EXCEPTION: WHO RECEIVES CARE, AND WHO DOES NOT?

In 2022, after the abortion ban became law in Ohio, the greatest urgency was determining who could still receive or not receive care. On paper, this should have been exactly my bailiwick—not just in my statewide leadership roles, but specifically as a high-risk obstetrician routinely managing patients with complicated pregnancies. However, it was not clear. Some questions in some states were straightforward as there were either explicit exceptions or prohibitions. For example, Ohio's ban had written exceptions for five conditions: preterm membrane rupture, bleeding, preeclampsia, diabetes, and multiple sclerosis. Alternatively, many states also had explicit prohibitions, and our ban likewise held no mercy for cases of rape, incest, fetal complications, or pregnant children. Between these two shorelines of clear exceptions and prohibitions, however, lie a vast ambiguous ocean of all other medical conditions, including, in Ohio, kidney disease, heart disease, and cancer. One of the fundamental problems with laws outlining specific exceptions is that it is impossible to encompass all existing diseases. For the totality of illnesses that were neither exemptions nor prohibitions, abortion was contingent upon a risk of death or "substantial and irreversible impairment of a major body function,"[1] but only then under the auspices of an affirmative defense.

What is an *affirmative defense*? It is a defense the accused is allowed to evoke, but in doing so they assume the burden of proof. Although varying from state to state, other classic examples of affirmative defense include insanity, entrapment, and acting in self-defense. For example, if I was accused of some crime and my defense was that I had not committed the act at all—if, say, I had an alibi showing that I was in another city—then the burden of proof lies upon the government to demonstrate that I had, in fact, committed the act. If instead I admit to the act itself but evoke an insanity defense, claiming that I had committed the act with an unsound mind, then the burden of proof falls upon me to prove insanity because insanity is affirmative. Most states, when drafting bans, elected to make abortion for maternal health—and even in some cases life itself—affirmative. Using our ban in Ohio as example, preeclampsia was a stated exception. If a physician provides an abortion to a patient with preeclampsia, therefore, in theory they should be immune from prosecution. If they are nevertheless charged, they should not be themselves responsible for the burden of proof. However, if they performed an abortion for a different condition not explicitly listed as an exception, such as if a patient had cancer, then they could, in theory, be criminally charged. Once charged, that doctor could evoke a defense of having acted to save a life, though saving a life would be an affirmative defense. The physician would assume the burden of proof that the patient's cancer necessitated abortion.

Some states right now have essentially no exceptions at all, with any abortions to save the parent falling under an affirmative defense. Confusingly, the word *exception* is often used by the public and media colloquially rather than with a formal meaning. It is often said that some states make exceptions for maternal life or health, when these are only covered by an affirmative defense without any formal exceptions at all.

As a society, we are also traversing entirely new territory absent prior case law, rulings, or precedent. Other affirmative defenses such as insanity, entrapment, or self-defense have long histories, with famous cases involving Twinkies, Patty Hurst, or reality shows starring Chris Hansen. These prior cases serve in turn as our guideposts and guardrails. But as of this writing, a physician has not yet evoked affirmative defense for maternal life or health. The most terrifying risks are those for which you do not know the underlying probabilities, what dice you may or may not hold in your hand. For example, physicians learn extensively about civil litigation, especially in litigious specialties such as high-risk obstetrics. Outcomes in lawsuits are notoriously unpredictable, though from years of case history we at least fundamentally know the parameters. We also knew and accepted those risks when we decided to enter medicine, when we selected our specialties. But we always imagined only civil litigation; we never foresaw the myriad other interactions with the legal system we now face.

Since Dobbs, for example, numerous OB-GYN physicians around the country have waded into our legal systems to stand against abortion bans as plaintiffs or in legislative matters. I was sued twice in 2023 in association with our reproductive freedom amendment, which is not as dramatic as it initially sounds. In Ohio, any ballot initiative technically consists of five citizens serving as "representatives of the petitioners." I was one of the five. Thereafter, if someone files a lawsuit against the "ballot amendment," the defendants formally include those five individuals. That was the case when antiabortion activists filed two such suits, both of which were subsequently dismissed by the Ohio Supreme Court. Unlike lawsuits in obstetrics, these entailed no damages or personal jeopardy; the issues at stake were nuances of constitutional processes rather than negligence.

One evening in 2023, strolling along green neighborhood sidewalks with our enormous St. Bernard, I realized I had not told my wife of the impending litigation.

"By the way," I tried to say casually, "a process server is coming to the house tomorrow with a summons. I believe someone will need to sign for it."

"You're being sued?"

"Yeah, but it's fine. I mean, it's quite serious because they're attempting to block the ballot initiative, but it is not medical, it's really sort of a technicality."

"But . . . there is a process server coming to our house tomorrow?"

The second time a summons arrived was on a Saturday, so I told the kids I was being sued again and we waited for the server, envisioning that classic scene from movies and TV. We were then disappointed when FedEx showed up; the summons only required a signature. It arrived in a thick manila envelope filled with papers ominously formal and dense with legalese, all of which was fundamentally bogus as in short order the court dismissed it unanimously. But these were lawsuits against ballot initiatives; criminal liability was something completely different.

Legally, obstetricians could not escape the myriad decisions surrounding pregnant patients with cancer or heart or kidney disease as they sat in our offices. A physician's role is to guide patients through the risks they face in order to make a choice. After Dobbs, this structure was often turned exactly on its head, with patients certain of their choice but the physicians now facing risks and not knowing what to do. The doctor could review the patient with counsel, describing the illness from their medical perspective, using medical terminology. The lawyer then could explain the legal thresholds for abortion, from the perspective of a lawyer using legal terminology. Yet even if they could harmonize perfectly, it may still not matter as an affirmative defense is contingent upon only future prosecutors, judges, or juries whose opinions are unknown.

Why not solve the problem of affirmative defense by having every state with a ban draw up a comprehensive list of exceptions that physicians could then simply follow? The immediate problem with this proposition is that, like the bans themselves, it fundamentally circumvents bodily autonomy in healthy patients. Envision, as a thought experiment, two patients seeking abortion, of whom only one could receive care. The first patient is pregnant with a life-limiting fetal genetic condition, while the second is completely healthy, but she is in her late teens and does not want to be pregnant. What would be the differing impacts of providing or refusing abortion care upon the total trajectory of these two patients' lives? Does one patient take precedence secondary to the fetal genetic condition alone?

Even if a list of exceptions is drawn, what does it include or exclude? There exist within the universe hundreds upon hundreds of diseases and conditions. For example, when Louisiana's abortion ban went into effect, the state released a list of twenty-four diagnoses for which physicians could provide abortion. The list came in the form of a declaration of emergency from the Department of Public Health, stating that "the Department of Health establishes the following exclusive list of anomalies, diseases, disorders, and other conditions that shall deem an unborn child 'medically futile' for purposes of [the new law]." The document then listed the twenty-four conditions, followed by a more open-ended twenty-fifth category of "a profound and irremediable congenital or chromosomal anomaly existing in the unborn child that is incompatible with sustaining life after birth,"[2] which required the certification of two physicians in their reasonable judgment.

Nancy Davis was a thirty-six-year-old woman living in Baton Rouge, Louisiana. In 2022, a routine ultrasound demonstrated *fetal acrania*, a condition in which the bones of the fetal skull are absent. Healthy brain development is impossible with acrania; the condition is incompatible with life. However, Louisiana's declaration of emergency had not listed acrania among the twenty-four diagnoses that would allow for abortion. First Davis was referred to a clinic that provided abortions, but after Dobbs, that clinic had already closed. She then requested abortion care from her hospital, but they declined because the declaration of emergency had not specifically listed acrania. There are literally hundreds of human diseases. Could the hospital have still provided abortion under Category 25, the more open-ended "profound and irremediable congenital or chromosomal anomaly"? Potentially, it could have. Perhaps a different physician or hospital may have braved providing care for Davis. But could a person be so certain of Category 25 that they would place themselves at criminal risk, and risk the potential loss of licensure and the end of their career? So they declined, with Davis later traveling out of state for abortion care.

Another problem with exceptions is that many diseases' risks exist along a continuum without clean demarcations along which to draw an arbitrary line. For example, physicians measure kidney disease by laboratory values such as serum creatinine or globular filtration rate (GFR), values that rise and fall with the disease severity. Pregnancy places a significant strain on the kidney, which many patients tolerate easily; for others, it throws them into renal failure, leading ultimately to dialysis and transplant waiting lists. For a pregnant patient in the first trimester, their future renal risks likewise rise and fall in accordance with their initial laboratory values. A maternal fetal specialist could have in their office two patients with chronic kidney disease, both early in the first trimester. The laboratory results of the first patient are only slightly worsened, indicating mild impairment, so the physician cites a low risk of pregnancy straining their kidneys into failure. The patient across the hall, meanwhile, has worse labs, so the physician cites a higher risk. In neither case is the outcome certain—the more severe patient may beat the odds, and the healthier patient may draw the bad straw—but both can approximate their odds from the laboratory values. Both can then make decisions regarding continuation or abortion. Counterintuitively, the patient with the worse disease will sometimes continue, already at peace with dialysis or transplantation as their likely future regardless of the pregnancy, while a patient with milder disease may be the most motivated to still preserve their long-term health and thus select abortion instead.

Now, when considering medical treatments and decisions, physicians must also weigh the legal risks to themselves. Where within this continuum of abnormal laboratory values does one draw a line and provide abortion care? Any laboratory value that is not completely normal? Or a value that is at least doubled? Or ten times worse? Any potential demarcation is arbitrary. Kidney disease is also just one disease among many that exist upon a similar continuum: the rising or falling blood sugars in diabetes, improving or worsening cardiac function in heart disease, or even the physical size of a pregnant child.

In July 2022, a pregnant ten-year-old came under the care of an Ohio ob-gyn. Public details are, appropriately, curtailed, though any pregnant ten-year-old is raped by definition as they cannot provide consent at that age. Authorities later caught the rapist, who entered a guilty plea in July 2023 and is currently serving a life sentence in our state. The legal process surrounding the rapist was quite clear: He had committed a grave crime, was charged, and was then sentenced through well-established procedures. But what of the doctor that day with the child in their office? What laws, legal history, processes, or precedent surrounded them?

We know from subsequent events that the family requested abortion care, though Ohio's ban cruelly made no exceptions for rape, children, or incest. The law did, however, allow abortion to protect maternal health, albeit under an affirmative defense. Carrying a pregnancy in a small ten-year-old body risks injury for obvious reasons of physical size. Visualize for a painful moment a ten-year-old at a full forty weeks gestation, struggling to stand from a chair or walk down a hall pulled under the weight of a term uterus: an image not only heartbreaking but clearly dangerous. But is the danger sufficient to qualify under an affirmative defense? At the time the child presented, no exact guidance in this regard existed, either within the law or from our state's attorney general. Although someone had taken time to exactly spell out a small number of exceptions, such as multiple sclerosis, this situation was unaddressed. Even if an answer existed for a ten-year-old, what then about the physical risks to a raped eleven-year-old? Would those also be qualifying? Does it matter if for any given age the girl is taller or shorter? The question, in all its grim literalness, is what size of a child's body is too small under the state's affirmative defense? Like rising and falling laboratory values or measures of heart or kidney function, the risk to children exists on a continuum in accordance with size.

Here we must pause to acknowledge the unequivocal horror of these questions. We would prefer to live our lives never thinking about raped children at all, let alone ponder which size body could safely carry a pregnancy to term. It is a subject for which cold, abstract contemplation is almost impossible, especially if you attempt to address it by imagining differing scenarios in your mind's eye.

In 2018, years before the Dobbs decision, one of our fellows training in MFM, along with a colleague and myself, statistically analyzed this exact question using the National Inpatient Sample, an enormous database of hospitalized patients from around the United States. We pulled the data on pregnancy outcomes in patients who were ten to fourteen years old, then later presented our results at the 2019 meeting of the American College of Obstetricians and Gynecologists.[3] I remember the fellow and I initially in my office discussing the possible project, how the subject matter made us deeply uncomfortable, a discomfort sufficient for us to question proceeding at all. However, if there exists an unanswered clinical question, the answer to which could inform future patient care, then the research should not just be contingent on our comfort. Ultimately, we found that pregnant children under fourteen years of age had significantly higher obstetric risks, including preeclampsia, than those between ages fourteen and eighteen, even when adjusted for other confounding factors.

The impulse to look away from terrible events is natural and understandable, though always also a decision we make. Imagine a reader seated at a table as their book transitions to the disquieting topic of pregnancy in small children. It would be entirely reasonable, if not in fact rational, to consider skipping ahead to the next chapter if this was a triggering topic. Presuming the reader is not a doctor nor a lawyer nor a legislator, they hopefully do not require a technical understanding of pregnancy in children anyhow. Each reader thus makes the free decision to continue or skip ahead. In the next building over, a pediatrics or obstetric trainee sits at a table as their medical textbook transitions to the disquieting topic of pregnancy in small children. Do they skip ahead to the next chapter? The subject is genuinely unsettling; however, they may the next day have a pregnant child walk into their office and will need to know what to do. Then in the next building, a group of legislators are crafting a bill to restrict abortion rights. Do they consider the disquieting subject of pregnancy in small children, or do they choose to metaphorically skip ahead? Does anyone in those meetings say: "I know this is unpleasant, but what guidance do we intend for a doctor when, tragically, though inevitably, a pregnant ten-year-old walks into their office?" I was not at those meetings in my state, but given the chaos that followed here it is clear there existed no functional plan. We wish children never to be victims of incest or rape, but we do not choose the world that exists—only what within that world we choose to see.

As is appropriate, I do not know which of our physicians saw the child that day, though after presumably weighing the facts and consulting lawyers, they decided not to risk abortion care. How did they tell the patient and her family? The decision must have been agonizing, and I would not judge or cast doubt on that physician; our legislators bear the sole responsibility for an essentially impossible bind. Perhaps we imagine ourselves more courageous, though I do not presume to know what I would have done myself. Regardless, the physician referred the child to neighboring Indiana, precipitating a complicated and ongoing chain of events, a story of courageous physicians facing their own personal risks.

Meanwhile, when the story first broke, our state attorney general appeared on a cable news program to raise suspicions. On July 11, he said "there was not a whisper of evidence"[4] that the raped ten-year-old had really existed. He said the story was "full of red flags." The story was completely true—the rapist identified and arrested shortly after that interview, the facts later confirmed in a court of law, the rapist now in prison. Of course, it was illogical for the case to have been doubted in the first place given the hundreds of children across the country who become pregnant annually from rape. The annual number of pregnant children at differing ages is also easily available for anyone bothering to examine public health records. The irresponsibility of questioning the story's truth was matched only by the irresponsibility of not having had a plan for this child already in place. The backlash and uproar were significant, our attorney general later stating that he believed the child would have qualified under affirmative defense.

After these events, ob-gyns now reasonably presume abortion care can be provided to a ten-year-old. But what about an eleven-year-old? Or a twelve-year-old? Or a ten-year-old in a different state with a different attorney general? These questions are neither hypothetical nor politically motivated to ensnare opponents into discomfort; pregnant eleven- and twelve-year-olds do walk into OB-GYN offices, and physicians genuinely do not know what to do.

When making these decisions in many restrictive states, however, physicians must only account for the physical risk to the small body of the child. What of the emotional aftermath of being forced to carry a pregnancy resulting from rape? The entire impact on their subsequent lives beyond the impact on their bodies themselves? In considering abortion under these bans, we must completely ignore these questions, as many of the laws are unconditionally without exceptions in this regard. But how does a physician actually do that? How many deeply held beliefs does this require we swallow down so hard against?

In the end, exceptions only masquerade as freedoms; they are in truth the crumbs of autonomy that legislators choose to bestow or withhold from us. We should not have to plead for exceptions. We should just have rights.

3 DECISION: WHAT IF YOUR DOCTOR IS NOT MAKING A DECISION?

After Dobbs, there was no question that patients would die as a result of the ruling. Less clear was who, where, and under what circumstances: A pregnant person with cancer, or worsening heart, lung, or kidney disease? Someone facing severe preeclampsia or hemorrhaging after an abruption? In the end, the true first death may be unknown. Although mortalities are now being publicly identified, they were likely preceded by others either unreported or in which the causative line between bans and mortality was more obscure. For example, completely healthy people who have normal pregnancies can rarely, though tragically, die from sudden delivery complications. Thus, the first person may have been medically unnotable but simply did not want to be pregnant and would have sought abortion if available, but due to being banned, quietly continued instead, later dying without national recognition. This is why, as meaningful epidemiologic data emerges in the years to come, it will be best to evaluate total mortality and abortion bans on a population level in addition to the stories of individuals. While awaiting more data, however, we are now seeing tragic individual stories.

ProPublica reported the death of Amber Thurman, a twenty-eight-year-old Georgia woman who presented with a uterine infection requiring a D&C procedure.[1] She was a single mother recently enrolled in nursing school who sought abortion after an unintended pregnancy. Although it was already illegal in Georgia, she drove to North Carolina instead, awakening at 4:00 a.m. for the long trip. Despite valiant efforts, she encountered traffic, arriving at the clinic a mere fifteen minutes late—and thus she was denied the procedure. She was provided with medication abortion instead, with the process to be completed back in Georgia. Complications such as incomplete tissue passage and uterine infections are uncommon after mifepristone, and when they do occur they are almost always resolved safely through a D&C procedure, with abortion exceedingly safe even after rare complications so long as patients can legally access care. Amber Thurman, however, never accessed her needed care.

On August 18, 2024, she presented to the Piedmont Henry Hospital Emergency Department in the suburbs outside of Atlanta with bleeding and infection. In many ways, her subsequent story parallels that of Porsha Ngumezi, another patient who bled to death in Houston. Both were in early pregnancy, both required a D&C to save their life, both sat in emergency departments instead deteriorating for hours upon hours without the procedure, until both ultimately descended far into critical illness. Both should be alive with their children today.

Why did they not receive D&Cs? In neither case have the hospitals or physicians involved provided detailed responses, and likewise we caution against speculating upon motivations or internal thought processes without complete information. We don't know what did or did not occur behind the scenes. For example, what if a physician had known the procedure was needed and had wanted to perform the D&C, but they encountered legal, administrative, or logistic barriers? Taking a patient to the operating room requires the agreement and cooperation of an entire cohort. What if an anesthesiologist or circulating nurse refused? Medical processes are not generally the act of a single individual but the collective efforts of many people in many roles, any one of whom can potentially stop the line if they raise concerns. Over the prior years, hospitals have, correctly, moved away from purely hierarchical structures to ones in which all employees are empowered to provide input and recommend changes. This restructuring improves patient safety and helps decrease medical error—though in cases in which abortion care is needed despite criminal bans, it also risks indeterminable delays.

Another contribution could have certainly been decision paralysis, which befalls physicians all too often. In both cases, the D&C procedure risked being interpreted as an illegal abortion. Although both states allow abortion, in theory, to save a life, the dangerous limitations of such defenses are reviewed throughout this book. A physician facing these scenarios could thus reasonably find themselves uncertain, falling into paralysis, unable to make a choice.

I have found myself in decision paralysis before. I am certain my wife has also, as has every physician at probably multiple points in their career. It is important for patients to recognize potential paralysis in their providers, especially with the new dangers faced after Dobbs. One of the disquieting aspects of decision paralysis is that you do not always realize you are in it at the moment. You believe instead that you are simply pondering the clinical question, pontificating over facts, awaiting more data, ideating rather than stagnating. Later, the paralysis is obvious in retrospect. But in the moment, you have to pull yourself out: Physicians need to make decisions.

Once, a patient stabbed in the chest arrived in the trauma bay, a Jane Doe found unresponsive with no identification, no one who knew her, no medical or obstetric records. All we could tell was that she appeared visually pregnant, though far from term, the uterus just rising above her belly button. She was unconscious and intubated, blood bubbling about the tube protruding from her mouth. While the trauma team descended upon her head and chest, we in obstetrics worked to first determine her weeks of gestational age. If the fetus was sufficiently mature to potentially survive if delivered—at that time, twenty-four weeks—then if she worsened, we might desperately perform a cesarean. *Perimortem cesareans* are those performed as the parent is about to die. Back then, we would or would not perform perimortem cesareans if the fetus was or was not at a sufficient number of weeks to survive, believing that otherwise the strain of surgery would only worsen a dire prognosis. Of note, modern practice has changed as we now recognize that cesareans above twenty weeks may improve rather than worsen outcomes in cardiac arrest independent of neonatal survival. In fact, such deliveries are increasingly referred to as *resuscitative cesareans*, emphasizing the primary intent of parental benefit.

An ultrasound was available in the trauma unit, though not specifically configured for obstetrics; it was used instead by surgeons evaluating kidneys, livers, and other organs, with settings, probes, and programing all different from our machines in labor and delivery. I started scanning; the fetus was still moving with cardiac activity, though obviously premature. But how premature? I needed to measure something, though if I was successful, I would only then have a raw number. The obstetric machines are programmed such that when you measure anything, an estimated gestational age appears automatically; for example, you measure the head or abdomen or femur, and in the corner of the screen the according number of weeks gestation appears. However, the trauma ultrasound only showed centimeters alone—and at that time I struggled to visualize anything at all, with the lights overhead brightened rather than darkened, the keypad unfamiliar, surgeons and nurses shouting back and forth. Then the patient's heart stopped beating.

Chest compressions commenced and difficult became almost impossible, with screen images now shifting up and down with CPR and only minutes left to perform or not perform a perimortem cesarean. Finally, a femur appeared, the bone comprising the top of the leg. I pressed freeze, then with the rollerball placed calipers on either end: two centimeters. Now I had a number, but with what gestational age did it correlate? If above twenty-four weeks, a perimortem cesarean was in order, but if under twenty-four weeks it was better to just allow the surgeons to work on the mother unimpeded. But at how many weeks was a femur two centimeters? I thought desperately. In the meantime, the team had assembled the surgical tray, betadine, and scalpel.

If I could freeze time, I could have carefully obtained every measurement to precisely determine the weeks of gestation. But all I had instead was two centimeters, a dying patient, and a team awaiting direction. I looked into my hand, trying to visualize a fetus with a two-centimeter femur, staring intently with my imagination, seeing if pediatrics could intubate what I saw if delivered. I stared and I stared.

"Are you doing a cesarean or not?" a resident yelled, pulling me out of the hypnosis into which I had fallen, standing there quietly among the chaos, just staring into my empty fingers. "No," I said, closing my hand. "She's too premature. Just do everything you can to save her." The trauma surgeon nodded. I wiped the ultrasound gel from her abdomen, and as I then stood watching, I can say with certainty they did everything they could.

What should patients do if they are concerned their physicians are lost in indecision? The simplest approach is to ask direct questions about their care. Why is a procedure being performed, or why not? If not performed, what would the indications for the procedure be? What future clinical changes would then trigger reconsideration? When undecided, physicians often gain clarity from vocalizing out loud; a situation becomes clear when we hear ourselves talking or having to provide justification, with the act of explanation itself breaking the spell. But as the patient you also need the exact picture, a plain understanding of rationale and next steps. For example, a patient in a restrictive state, previable with severe preeclampsia, bleeding, or prematurely ruptured membranes, should ask if an abortion would be offered and receive a straightforward answer.

Doctors dislike delivering bad news, though after years of training we still disburse medical information without hesitancy. I deliver terrible diagnoses usually multiple times a week. But alternatively, a doctor may be reluctant to disclose that a needed procedure cannot be legally or administratively provided, with this new scenario foreign and deeply disquieting. Or perhaps they themselves made the decision to not assume criminal risks and are now struggling with shame. Then, rather than a straightforward disclosure, the doctor's discomfort may instead yield embarrassment and guilt, all in turn giving birth to delay and obfuscation. Or perhaps the physician is advocating for the procedure, but they must keep appealing upward through legal and administrative layers, conceptualizing themselves as progressing while, in actuality, time is running out, with the patient only descending further into sepsis or hemorrhage. But if a patient cannot receive a procedure from a given physician in a given hospital in a given state, it is critical that they receive this information clearly and expediently. Thus, the need under abortion bans is for patients to ask direct questions and physicians to provide translucent answers in response. If a patient cannot receive a needed procedure, the patient needs to know. Even if the doctor cannot believe the words emanating from their mouth, cannot believe the situation we are in—even if the doctor is themselves responsible, patients need to know. They need to know if they are endangered, if they need to leave, find another hospital, or escape the state entirely. They need to know if now is the time to fight for their own lives.

Hospitalized patients and loved ones can also ask if their facility permits a family-initiated rapid response (FIRR). The exact systems for codes and medical emergencies, as well as the types of responses, will vary from hospital to hospital with differing criteria of endangerment and activation. Traditionally, emergency alarms are sounded by medical personnel. However, there is a growing trend of allowing patients and loved ones to trigger emergency responses as well. Thus, if a person believes they or a partner is worsening, that a situation is becoming emergent and care needs to be escalated, a FIRR can be called and an emergency support team will arrive at the bedside.

Of course, sometimes it is the physicians who are certain and the patients who are undecided. Or perhaps doctors have presented the patient with two options from which they must choose, with the patient then falling into paralysis instead. Like I have faced indecision as a physician, I have also experienced indecision as a support person.

My wife and I were in fellowship at the University of Pittsburgh when we had our first child. Although technically still in training, we had been in medicine for years, long enough to have seen patients make choices hundreds of times, but we had never actually had to make medical decisions ourselves.

We had our first ultrasound around twelve weeks, and I immediately saw the ovarian mass on the screen. It was larger than the fetus—larger, in fact, than the entire uterus, about ten centimeters in its widest dimension. In gynecology, we classify ovarian cysts as simple or complex; a *simple cyst* is one that is just filled with fluid, like a water balloon. This cyst was not simple. It had septations. Flecks of debris floated about on ultrasound. Although cancer was statistically improbable at my wife's age, we also could not technically rule it out given the mass's size and concerning appearance.

The basic decision was if a surgeon should remove the mass during the pregnancy itself or after delivery. There were risks to both approaches. If removed during pregnancy, the surgery would be timed for about the middle, striking a balance between the risks of the first trimester and those of the third when the expanding uterus mechanically makes removal difficult or impossible. Of note, just performing surgery in pregnancy in and of itself is surprisingly safe. For example, if a patient breaks a bone and needs an orthopedic procedure performed upon a limb, medications can be selected that are appropriate for the fetus, and just having anesthesia, undergoing some surgery, and then waking back up carries almost no risk specific to the pregnancy. What would pose risk in our case was the surgeon physically entering the abdominal cavity itself. It would be difficult to remove the mass without also touching or manipulating the uterus with our growing fetus inside. There would be a small though present risk of preterm labor, pregnancy loss, or other complications.

What if, instead, my wife decided against surgery during pregnancy? The mass still needed to be removed eventually; it was 10 centimeters and complex. But that could happen in the postpartum period after delivery was safely over. Most likely, the mass would just be there, asymptomatically hanging out through the pregnancy; if we had never seen it on ultrasound, we would never have been the wiser. It would shift and squeeze as it accommodated the growing uterus, but despite its large size, nothing bad would happen. That is what would be most probable, but not what was certain. A mass this large could also precipitate emergent complications. It might not tolerate the pressure of the expanding uterus and could rupture, bleeding and spilling its liquid contents into my wife's abdomen. It could also undergo torsion (torse). *Ovarian torsion*, similar to testicular torsion in males, is when an ovary twists such that it kinks off its own blood supply. Torsion is often caused by a cyst on the ovary that then moves it around, including when shifted about by an expanding uterus in pregnancy. The sensation of torsion is reported to be similar between males and females and likely feels like an injury to the scrotum: a pain that is sickening in nature, often accompanied by intense nausea and vomiting.

If a person had a crystal ball and knew the ovarian mass would cruise through the pregnancy without complications, then they would leave it alone until after delivery. There would be no reason to assume the risk of abdominal surgery in mid-pregnancy. However, if the crystal ball said that the mass was going to rupture or torse, then they would schedule the removal for well before that happened.

Of course, there is no crystal ball, but we do know that the chance of rupture or torsion increases as the size of the mass increases. Thus, for a mass that is small, the risk is low, and a doctor would recommend not removing it mid-pregnancy. You could still end up with rupture or torsion, but the probability is less than the risks of scheduled surgery. On the other hand, if the mass is large, then the chances are higher, and you would assume the risk of removing it mid-pregnancy. So potentially, you can make decisions just in accordance with size. But at what size do the scales tilt? As is often the case, the medical literature has conflicting results, though a rough answer is around 10 centimeters. In other words, we were right at the tipping point. There was not a clear, obvious answer. Thus, like the hundreds of patients we had seen in the past and would see in the future, we had to make a decision.

We met formally with my own MFM attending. We pulled the research papers ourselves; my wife and I read them around our dining room table. We talked about the potential surgery. We talked about the risks if we left the mass in place. We took our dogs for walks through Frick Park and the brick streets of Regent Square, then later hot dogs at D's. Weeks went by. But eventually decisions are always made for you.

One early Sunday morning, when my wife was still just at seventeen weeks, she awoke suddenly doubled over in pain, sickeningly nauseous. I had seen this several times as a physician. It was ovarian torsion. The cyst had been moving in my wife's abdomen as the uterus grew, and now was positioned such that it had kinked off the blood supply. Without blood flow, the tissue of the cyst was starting to die and soon would necrose. Having an abdomen flooded with 10 centimeters of dead, necrotic ovarian mass not only would cause intense pain, but could also cause her to become critically ill.

I called my colleague and drove my wife to the hospital. The emergent surgical incision ran vertically all the way from her belly button to the bottom of her abdomen. My colleague had to almost impossibly balance speed and caution, quickly removing the mass while also not disturbing the adjacent uterus with the fetus inside. If you add the fact that this was the wife of her fellow, and a fellow herself, I am not sure if I myself have ever done or will do anything as stressful. I still regularly see this colleague at the large, annual meetings of our professional organization, the Society for Maternal-Fetal Medicine. Several times, I have thanked her for saving my wife and son that day, usually proclaimed somewhat drunkenly at the bar around one or two in the morning. We laugh, and she makes some statement about how stressful it all was.

The mass was successfully removed. The pregnancy continued. In pregnancy, wound healing after abdominal surgery is complicated by the incision being continually stretched atop the expanding uterus while trying to close. Eventually, my wife went back to work. Managing pediatric cancer can be weighty without also either being pregnant or recovering from surgery—or, in her case, both. Unfortunately, even though everything went well, patients after abdominal surgery are predisposed to preterm labor in the weeks that follow.

My wife went into labor a little after thirty-four weeks while at work. My son ended up spending about two weeks in the neonatal intensive care unit (NICU) before coming home with us in good health. Years later, he is a teenager a bit taller than me, and he is at the University of Pittsburgh now, a student rowing for the crew team. While he was still in the NICU through those first two weeks, I went back to work so that I could take my paternity leave once he was actually home and I could be of the most use. On those days, I would work in labor and delivery and then, when my shift was done, ride the elevator down to the NICU and visit him in his warmer. Sometimes I would swing by during lunch if things were not too busy. Working in high-risk obstetrics, I would often see my own patients down in the NICU who I had delivered in the prior days or weeks. This was before most NICUs had only private rooms, so the bassinets and incubators were all in rows throughout a large open unit with rocking chairs in between. The other parents would take their kids out of their warmers and I would take out mine, and we would all sit rocking back and forth. During those two weeks, we delivered quadruplets; a day later, when I went to visit my son, four other new warmers were lined up around him.

The ovarian cyst torsed prior to us having made a decision about surgery; we remained undecided until the end. But indecision is always the decision to continue unabated; reading and rereading the book chapter on ovarian masses eventually becomes itself the decision not to have surgery. Not performing surgery, of course, would have also been a reasonable choice, as the ovary ultimately torsing was not at the time a forgone inevitability. But in that case, I would have optimally had a clear opinion against surgery. This is true not only for physicians and patients but throughout life, including in the political and legislative choices we are making right now.

After the Dobbs decision, Ohioans knew we needed to bring a reproductive ballot measure before voters, but we had to choose the year. Ours is one of the few states that allow for voter-initiated amendments in odd-numbered years, other states requiring instead alignment with major senatorial or federal elections. So in 2022, we could either move quickly toward 2023 or plan further ahead into 2024. Both years held stark advantages and disadvantages, debated widely at the time. Choosing 2023 felt too soon; it would require organization and coalition building at a breakneck speed. In addition, the electorate in off-cycle elections tends to be demographically older and more conservative. However, 2024 held risks as well. Multiple states limited to even-numbered years would likely advance initiatives in 2024, meaning that Ohio would be competing nationally for attention and resources. A 2024 campaign would also be more expensive as we would be purchasing commercials and advertising amid a presidential and senatorial election. The stakes of the decision were terrifying as we knew there would only be one generational shot at the ballot box. So there was debate and more debate. But what if we remained persistently uncertain? Indecision would eventually become the decision for 2024.

Rather than oscillating endlessly, we instead leapt forward into 2023. I wish I could say I had been brave myself in this regard, but the credit for this decision goes to others—in particular, the physician leaders of Ohio Physicians for Reproductive Rights (OPRR). And what would have been the human cost of waiting until 2024? We would have likely remained under our ban during that time—patient after patient, day after day, denied care while we pondered and strategized. Right now, we all have to make ourselves make decisions—because they are never not made, just eventually made by events rather than by us.

4 EXPERTISE: HOW DO WE IDENTIFY EXPERTISE?

Years ago, when I was a new intern, we had a patient with chronic hepatitis C who had just delivered that morning. When she arrived on the postpartum floor, she asked for help breastfeeding, horrifying the nurse, who stated that breastfeeding was contraindicated due to the baby's risk of contracting hepatitis C through breastmilk. The patient explained that it was perfectly safe, as she had investigated breastfeeding with the virus extensively beforehand. The nurse disagreed. Everything then spiraled rapidly, with the patient insisting on breastfeeding, the nurse insisting it was unsafe, the patient demanding her baby, and the nurse instead rolling the bassinet down the hall to the nursery. The patient followed despite her postpartum state; the nurse closed the nursery door, the patient asked to call the manager, the nurse said she would call security, and the patient said she was going home to call the police.

Upstairs in my call room, the pager alarmed. I was told a patient was leaving the hospital despite having just delivered an hour or two earlier. As discharge this early is never recommended, I needed her to sign paperwork acknowledging this action as "against medical advice." That was all the information given to me over the phone: no hepatitis C, no breast feeding, no security, no baby held behind a closed nursery door with discord erupting outside. Thus, I emerged unprepared into the scene of a furious patient, a furious nurse, an authoritative manager, and a security officer who appeared deeply uncomfortable with everything occurring around him. As soon as I entered, everyone asked me the same question at once: Is it safe to breastfeed with hepatitis C?

The nursing station was now silent awaiting my reply. I didn't know. I racked my brain. I was a new intern and had not yet had a patient with hepatitis C who wanted to breastfeed. In medicine there are just . . . so many facts.

After what felt like an hour, I almost whispered, "I don't know." The weary patient roughly signed the discharge forms, walked over to hand me the crumpled papers, then looked into my eyes, stating, "You are an idiot. I am going home and calling a lawyer." She then walked out through the heavy automatic doors. As soon as she left, I ran upstairs to the call room where we kept the obstetric textbooks. This was before wireless internet and smartphones allowed you to instantly access any needed fact at any given second. The textbook was *Gabbe's Obstetrics*, the second edition, with the dark blue cover and stylized drawings of fetuses on the front. I looked up "hepatitis C" in the index, then flipped through thick swaths of pages to finally read that breastfeeding with hepatitis C is perfectly safe. Although there are many maternal viruses that risk transmission through breastfeeding, HIV being a classic example, hepatitis C has never been detected in breastmilk. The patient had been absolutely correct.

After I picked up the phone and called my attending physician, I had some time to reflect. Although I had studied so hard through four years of medical school, there were so many things about medicine that I still didn't know. There exist in the world legions of differing viruses, bacteria, and parasites, each with different clinical presentations, geographic topographies, and treatments. There are hundreds of drugs with differing indications and side effects. Any organ in the body can transform into not one but many different variants of cancer, each of which then often have unique staging systems. The obstetric textbook I held in the call room that day was heavy in my hands, hundreds of pages in length. Medical knowledge is like an ocean you attempt to drink during medical school. Then, during your first year of internship, you repetitively confront—like I did that day—all your knowledge gaps that persist despite your four years of study.

In November 2019, HR 413, an all-encompassing antiabortion bill, was introduced to the Ohio state legislature. It was 723 pages long and mandated swaths of new regulations, ranging from defining fertilized eggs as "unborn children" to outlining a crime of "abortion murder." I presume it reflected many hours of work for some combination of legislators, lawyers, and aids. Among the bill's cosponsors was State Representative John Becker, well-known for extreme views on reproduction, if not medicine writ large. For example, the following year, he requested that a state appeals court order the arrest of our Republican governor for alleged crimes, including terrorism, related to our COVID-19 public health measures.[1] He also earlier that year sponsored house bill 182, which included language on "ectopic reimplantation." Ectopic gestations occur when a blastocyst implants in a location other than the normal interior of the uterus, most often the fallopian tube. Once implanted, relocation is impossible; an embryo cannot be simply disengaged and reimplanted in the uterus like a gardener repotting a plant. Likewise, a gestation in the fallopian tubes will usually continue growing until it ruptures in a life-threatening hemorrhage. The dangers cannot be understated: Ectopic gestations are a leading cause of death for pregnant patients. Despite that, there exist fringe individuals who believe reimplantation to be possible either currently or sufficiently near in the future as to warrant mandating the procedure now. Specifically, Representative Beker had included such language previously in another submission. Thus, when I received the PDF of the new bill, I typed "ectopic" into the search bar and there it was: "A physician must . . . takes all possible steps to preserve the life of the unborn child, while preserving the life of the woman. Such steps include, if applicable, attempting to reimplant an ectopic pregnancy into the woman's uterus."[2]

I took a screenshot, added snarky comments about how this was impossible, sent a tweet, and was shortly catapulted into the weird world of *going viral*.[3] HB 413 quickly became, with complete justification, a national laughingstock, the entirety of its 723 pages sunk by the consummate idiocy of lines 5377 and 5378. Despite an antiabortion majority in our legislature, it was never granted even a courtesy hearing, dying an ignoble death in committee.

During the fiasco, I could not help but ponder the gulfs that exist between physicians and many legislators: the years upon years we study through medical school, residency, and fellowship relative to those crafting legislation despite no medical training at all. But in addition to medical knowledge, humility is also important, the understanding of what one may not know in addition to what we do. Beyond expertise itself, to what extent are laws even given thought or contemplation?

Later in an interview, Representative Becker was asked why ectopic reimplantation had been included in the now failed bill: "I heard about it over the years," Becker said. "I never questioned it or gave it a lot of thought."[4]

But how do you identify medical expertise? Not just legislators, but the public, the media, and, most importantly, patients themselves? This is a critical modern question as we are living in an era of bountiful, often unregulated misinformation, which in turn directly impacts patients' lives. For example, you can draw an essentially straight line between not believing in and not receiving a measles vaccination and dying from measles. But for those seeking medical guidance in good faith, how do they navigate this landscape? Normally, we would turn to our leaders, to our state and federal institutions, to physicians themselves. However, these sources may now be unreliable, with many legislators and even prominent doctors increasingly misinformation's champions rather than its combatants—particularly in questions of reproductive health, and especially under abortion bans.

What if tomorrow I suddenly, magically became a legislator myself? Hopefully, as a physician, I would be placed on a health committee where I could craft laws and ask informed questions during hearings. But the next day, the chamber could gather to debate the budget, then a tax bill, then the highway bill. I listen in my chair as a civil engineer speaks on subjects for which I have no expertise but nevertheless will be voting upon later that day. It is commonly stated that legislators are not physicians, though on any other day they may also not be bankers, educators, farmers, business owners, or law enforcement agents. Lake Erie forms the long northern border of our state, and thus our representatives may vote upon matters of ecology, water quality, and shipping. As an imaginary legislator, how would I vote regarding our Great Lake?

Every governing body has publicly available schedules, bills, and hearings that, as a thought experiment, you can freely peruse while imagining yourself as the legislator. What would you do in that role? No one person can have expertise in everything, but sometimes more important than our own expertise is the recognition of our limits and how to then find and trust the expertise of others. For physicians working in primary care—for example, in family medicine—these decisions are a central and daily aspect of their jobs. For each patient, at each visit, they must decide when they are comfortable managing the patient themselves and when instead to refer the patient to specialists. In MFM, I am in this same scenario as my patients are often pregnant concurrently with some other unrelated disease. Which of my pregnant patients with lupus, heart disease, or thyroid disorders do I or do I not refer to rheumatology, cardiology, or endocrinology versus managing them myself? Through my career, I have moved into administrative and advocacy positions in which I maintain this collaborative model, with my goal to always remember where my expertise as a physician ends and respect within their bailiwick the expertise of others. For legal matters, I follow the advice of counsel; for legislative matters, policy experts; for media appearances, my communication directors. Sometimes doctors in advocacy positions will justifiably rail against legislators making medical decisions, then later disagree with their pollsters on polling or with lawyers on the law.

But how do you then find the best consultants or know whom to trust? Often it is straightforward. For my complicated patients, there exist the other specialists on our faculty. For hospital or professional organizations, you are directed to specific staff. But what if I am again the imaginary legislator, sitting in a chair, listening to a stream of conflicting experts on highways or waterways? Two engineers might take turns at the lectern while presenting diametric opinions. Or what if I am a patient facing disparate recommendations from two individuals—both doctors, both clad in long white coats?

There is, of course, no perfect answer. The subject itself could easily fill an entire book, if not the philosophic branch of epistemology. But I find that one of the best and simplest approaches for patients and physicians alike is to just try to avoid genetic errors.

What is a *genetic error*? Once when I was a resident, I had to present at conference a patient who had battled ovarian cancer for years. Her original surgery was almost six years in the past, after which she had been in remission, then suffered a recurrence, then entered remission again, but now had new metastases. Preparing for the next day's presentation, I sat down in front of her multiple large manila charts, opened the first page of her first chart, and—well, she did not have ovarian cancer. She had endometrial cancer. The initial surgery had been for endometrial cancer, later confirmed by pathology, but then at some point in the following years it was transcribed as ovarian in a single note via simple human error. But like a genetic mutation progressing through family trees, the mistake was then replicated over and over through the subsequent records. The following morning, I stood with the stack of charts before the committee gathered in the conference room, specialists from an array of fields prepared to debate the treatment of recurrent ovarian cancer. "So . . . ," I started awkwardly. "Our first patient has endometrial cancer."

In the field of logic, a *genetic fallacy* occurs when someone judges an assertion on its origin rather than its merits—that is, on the *genesis* of the notion. There are two types of genetic fallacies: first are the *affirmative fallacies* in which you believe trusted sources without verification, and second are the negative fallacies in which you erroneously reject premises from the untrusted. For that cancer patient, each subsequent patient note believed without verification the one that had preceded it, thus propagating the mistake. Ideally, we would assess all of life's assertions independently from their sources. If I find an individual whose beliefs, experiences, and worldview all differ from my own, and they tell me that today it will rain, I would optimally still pack an umbrella. If I make an assertion to a legislator who opposes abortion, I will hope it will not then be dismissed instantly at its source. Likewise, I caution to avoid negative fallacies when interacting with individuals holding disparate views.

Once I was walking with colleagues through the state legislature, going from office to office while lobbying on behalf of our profession and patients. As we turned a corner down the hall, a team member warned us that the next politician was a clown. That is unfortunate, I thought; our purpose that day was quite serious. I braced myself for an adversarial encounter. I was already nervous as they were known to vote against abortion rights. But then my associate clarified that their expression had been literal rather than an insinuation of character; the legislator, to their credit, was a volunteer clown who performed for children to raise money for pediatric charities.

They were dressed that day in normal business attire, though walking into the office we could see a mix of the usual political tchotchkes—pins, posters, the legislator in framed photos cohorting with the famous—and then clown paraphernalia: curly rainbow hair atop a white wig block, a bright round nose, flower lapels, and elongated red shoes sitting near the conference table. I looked about wondering what sequence of life choices had led me to this place. Then we sat at the table, with me hoping that none of us would proceed into genetic fallacy.

The weeks heading into our 2023 vote on the reproductive freedom amendment saw a typhoon of commercials for and against the measure. Among the opposition arguments was the specter of full-term surgical abortions in healthy patients. Stories were told after the amendment of women at "nine months" without complications being able to easily request an abortion, which doctors would oblige; the procedure was then described graphically. Often this information's genesis was in sources that appeared otherwise credible: our state's political leaders, with nicely combed hair and airs of certainty. A letter circulated by the Archdiocese of Cincinnati stated: "The amendment provides caveats such that a healthy, fully formed infant in the womb who otherwise could be delivered with no issues would still be a candidate for a surgical dismemberment abortion."[5] A former US president in a TV commercial proclaimed that in the "ninth month" physicians are allowed to "rip the baby out of the womb of the mother."[6]

Such assertions were fantastical. Although abortions in the third trimester are uncommonly performed, there has never been a known procedural abortion in a healthy, full-term pregnancy. The amendment explicitly did not permit such procedures—and even if they were somehow legal, no physician would simply do that as we are not murderous caricatures. The subsequent national 2024 election cycle, however, felt even worse with frequent discussion of abortions somehow occurring after the delivery. On the most basic level, this is impossible as abortion is the discontinuation of a pregnancy, so any events that occur after delivery would never be an *abortion* by the definition itself. For example, a *stillbirth* is defined as the loss of a fetus prior to delivery. Thus, if a child was born, then a day or two after the delivery passed away, nobody would ever describe these sad events as a stillbirth, because that is just not the definition of a stillbirth. It would be a *neonatal death*. Likewise, the concept of an abortion occurring after delivery is nonsensical.

When political leaders talk about abortion "after delivery," they are likely confabulating perinatal palliative care, in which a delivery is performed in the context of a life-limiting fetal condition, with the goals of maximizing comfort and paternal bonding rather than prolonging life. The nuances of these situations are both complicated and critical, the decisions often painful, but these are not abortions—especially as described grotesquely by pundits in front of adulating crowds.

Ultimately, in 2023, our state amendment was successful despite the misinformation, and since then none of our opponents' reckless prophecies have actually come to pass. But prior to the election, legions believed authoritative figures' loud but fallacious proclamations. We can feel right now as if genetic fallacies are everywhere we look—and in theory, the populace should be able to trust their leaders without trepidation. We should be able to believe the statements of an American president or state attorney general. We should be able to trust the Food and Drug Administration or the Centers for Disease Control and Prevention (CDC). But now even doctors are no longer uniformly trustworthy, with fringe physicians regularly appearing in legislative testimony, at courtroom lecterns, and on podcasts. What do we do when we cannot even be sure of trusting doctors?

Many years ago, my wife and I participated in two medical trips to Nicaragua with a wonderful nonprofit organization. The second summer that we were there, a local gynecologist I had worked with the year before requested my help with a hysterectomy. The exact surgical indication was lost to my limited Spanish, but he needed help as the patient was in her seventies. In light of her age, the anesthesiologist had only agreed to a spinal, in which a single dose of anesthetic solution is injected into the spinal column. The medication then numbs the patient under the level of injection. Relative to other approaches, a spinal often carries the lowest risk as the patient remains fully awake, but it has the danger of eventually wearing off, similar to a dentist injecting lidocaine: It initially numbs your mouth, but later your mouth returns to normal. Speed is thus critical when operating under a spinal, lest the patient regain sensation while still open. Therefore, he requested my help, believing we could work best together: he on one side of the table and me on the other, two sets of hands moving quickly, entering the abdomen, performing the hysterectomy, then getting back out before the anesthetic wore off.

The following morning, we met at the hospital entrance, and he led me down the halls to the surgical suite. He introduced me to the patient, and I stumbled through a brief conversation. She made few expressions, as is typical when suppressing a well of anxiety; she was certainly in no mood to entertain an American's attempted Spanish. She wore a plain hospital gown, and her long, grey hair was held back with a tie. I wondered what she may have experienced over her decades in Nicaragua: the civil war, Daniel Ortega, the Contras.

The operating room had lime-green walls lit by fluorescent lights. Seated on the table, the patient arched her bare, thin back, then winced as the anesthesiologist slid the needle between two vertebrae, injected the anesthetic fluid, and laid her flat as the nurse washed her abdomen. The gynecologist, surgical assistant, and I scrubbed, then entered through hinged doors to don gowns and gloves. The air was thick with humidity, all the more stifling when you are also wrapped in blue cloth gowns. Setting the sterile drape, I noticed an existing horizontal scar across her abdomen, obviously surgical in nature. I realized I did not really know her medical history, as I had not spoken with her myself and the chart was written in Spanish. The assistant erected her rectangular stand filled with metal instruments, then handed the gynecologist a scalpel. He made his incision overtop the existing scar, after which we descended efficiently and systemically together through anatomic layers: the skin, the adipose tissue, the abdominal fascia, the membranous peritoneum, and then finally the abdominal cavity itself, obscured initially by the large and small bowel progressively packed away behind moistened white pads as we moved further toward the uterus. When we entered the anatomic pelvis, however, we did not see the uterus. Perhaps it was just smaller or located more distally as postmenopausal patients often have prolapse. But we continued not to see anything as we delved deeper until we came upon the vagina itself, cleanly incised across the top then long ago sutured closed; the patient had already had a hysterectomy. The uterus was no longer present, the entire surgery a dangerous mistake.

The surgeon and I looked for a second down into the pelvis. Then the assistant looked also, made a startled exclamation, and began speaking rapidly. The surgeon replied, haltingly at first, then more forcefully, the two now arguing back and forth, with the anesthesiologist and nurse joining in as well. They were talking too fast for me to catch most words, but I knew exactly what they were saying. One by one the gynecologist pulled out the white pads securing the bowels, loops of intestine sliding back into the space where there once was a uterus, then asked for the fascial suture to close the abdominal wall. I asked a question, and he gruffly replied that I could leave now, so I stepped away from the table, pulling off my gown, my scrubs underneath sweat drenched from the humidity; everyone in the operating room was still arguing heatedly. As I began to exit, I saw the patient at the head of the table and remembered that with the spinal anesthetic, she was completely awake, listening to everything now shouted around her.

I stepped through the hospital doors into the sun outside, my unease contrasting with the bright and brilliant landscape about me. How could a mistake that fundamental have occurred? This elderly patient was now going to spend days recovering from a meaningless surgery. Was the local physician just confused or misinterpreted the preexisting scar? Or, more hauntingly, was the patient also unaware, with a hysterectomy performed upon her in the past without knowledge or consent? Regardless of the source, I had made a genetic error; I had accepted the gynecologist's assertion without additional clarification. Walking back to the clinical building, I constructed reasonable arguments for why this was not my fault. My medical Spanish, for example, is not fluent; my time with the patient before the surgery had been brief. However, though genetic errors may, in retrospect, be explainable, they are also always still choices that we make. I not only chose to accept the physician's first assertion, but I then made additional choices along the way. I did not request details of the surgery's indication. I did not inquire into imaging studies or the source of her prior scar. My Spanish had certainly been adequate to have asked these basic questions, but I chose not to.

When someone accepts false assertions about reproductive health, they are also making choices. There exists no default requirement for anyone to believe anything. Not only do we freely adopt or reject the assertions we encounter through life, but more foundationally we adopt our original framework of belief, freely select the lens through which we view the world. We choose our required levels of evidence, our thresholds for the adoption of precepts. Even before genetic errors, we choose which channels to watch for news, which websites to visit. We are not swept passively into misinformation, tricked through sleight of hand or magical spells. In 2019, when Ohio's HR 413 included nonsensical language about ectopic reimplantation, this was how it had been chosen to be written.

For the immediate future, my practical recommendation for sources to look to for reproductive guidance would be our medical professional organizations, the country's varying specialty and subspecialty societies and colleges. Such institutions are independent of our federal government and thus, unlike former stalwarts such as the CDC, are immutable to election outcomes or changes in leadership. For example, when the CDC recently removed broad swaths of critical guidelines from its websites, the American College of Obstetricians and Gynecologists chose to host the recovered information online instead. Increasingly, other organizations also have public-facing information and patient recommendations, all of which in theory should weather the years to come. But are even these organizations infallible? Certainly, searching through the past, you can easily uncover prior recommendations that were later found to be incorrect, if not problematic.

More fundamentally, pointing to sources that are currently trustworthy fails to resolve the problem of genetic fallacies; it is in fact antithetical to the fallacy itself. Instead, perhaps we would be better served by reexamining our *epistemic thresholds*, the degrees of evidence we require to adopt a belief. What would I do as the imagined legislator before two engineers debating bridges, a subject about which I know essentially nothing? First, I would strive to avoid genetic errors, try to disregard the engineer's political affiliation, appearance, or demographic similarities. But then I would need to weigh their arguments against my threshold for belief. What evidence does each present, what prior research? Do they tell stories that are dramatic, though also likely idiosyncratic? Or do they present a more overarching narrative? Do their recommendations apply specifically to the bridges in my state? A binary choice faces me at the end of the session, because regardless of my own knowledge of support beams, buttresses, or cantilevers, I am going to have to cast a vote. The same is true of our patients, who, regardless of their own medical backgrounds, need to make decisions after we finish talking. So, what are the frameworks we will choose to adopt, and how tightly will we hold onto them in the years to come?

5 CONSENT: WHAT IF WE HELD PHYSICIANS AND LEGISLATORS TO SIMILAR STANDARDS?

In November 2020, I served as a poll worker during the COVID-19 pandemic. Due to the virus, there were concerns about having sufficient election workers for the wheels of democracy to turn smoothly. I had not yet received the vaccine, so the risk of a long day facing incoming crowds was not insignificant. I wore my mask tightly, repetitively sanitized, and ate my packed lunch seated away from the others. We gave each voter a small, disposable rubber sheath to roll over their finger for the touchscreens—basically a finger condom, the humor of which waned after the first hour.

The atmosphere was tense, with the weight of a federal election mixed with the hovering danger of COVID. We gathered the night before at the church that would serve as the polling place, where our station manager reviewed the steps for the following morning. Speed and efficiency were essential to open for the earliest voters on their way to work: setting tables and registration areas, posting the required signs, erecting booths, and powering on scanners. But among the first actions that following morning was the one I most wanted to be assigned: planting the American flag in its designated location outside. This was the task heaviest in symbolism: the flag, our precious emblem of democracy, the very American values for which we were about to risk ourselves against a deadly viral pandemic.

We gathered the following morning around 5:00 a.m. As soon as we began dividing roles, I asked the manager if I could place the flag. "Sure," she said, handing me a flag the size of a placemat on a wooden stake around three feet in length, reminding me of the exact location it should be placed.

I walked out through the doors into the cold November air, pulsing with energy despite the vast silence of the early hour, with the sky still full of stars as I strolled to the designated point. I then straightened to dramatically thrust the stake into the ground—but the underlying earth was firmer than anticipated, my degree of force poorly calibrated, and the wooden flagpole broke apart.

I stood there for a moment, stricken, beholding the flag and the pieces of fractured tan wood in my hands. With no other option, I slumped back to the building where the manager was busy pointing and directing the other workers to hang signs and set up machines. "I . . . ah . . . I broke the flag."

"You did what?" She turned to see the broken pole in my hand, the other workers pausing to come gawk as well. "Yeah," I said. "I think I pushed too hard, and the ground was firmer than I thought and . . ."

"We don't have time for this." She exclaimed, reaching into a bag and pulling out a collection of smaller flags. She handed them to another, presumably more competent worker, asking her to plant them instead.

After that, I was trusted with only the most menial jobs. I lifted heavy bags of paper ballots onto tables. I stood outside and pointed toward the building's entry when voters approached, looking out upon the cluster of smaller flags in the grass a few yards away. Throughout the day I was the butt of friendly jokes, other folks ribbing me to take care not to break anything else as they walked by. I did not know any of the other workers; nobody knew or would have presumed that I was a doctor or university faculty. For people who do not already know me, I often suspect that my first impression is that of a burly stuttering oaf—likely harmless, but also possibly missing a lightbulb or two upstairs. Thankfully, I am a better physician than poll worker, two jobs with little in common except perhaps that medicine and democracy both lie upon a bedrock of consent.

On that November day, voters expressed their consent in our government, and every day, patients in our offices express consent in their care. Be it explicit or implied, direct or through a guardian, nothing in medicine proceeds without consent. Likewise, the wheels of government turn with the consent of the governed. For both institutions, however, this has not always been the case; our history is replete with medical, physical, and legislative consent violations, from our nation's founding onward. One infamous example from medicine is Dr. Marion Sims, a pioneer of gynecologic surgery and namesake of medical instruments such as the Sims speculum. As is devastatingly detailed in the 2023 book *Say Anarcha* and elsewhere, Dr. Sims crafted his surgical techniques by operating upon enslaved Black women without consent or anesthesia, the magnitude of physical pain from which is difficult to fathom. Many of the names of those operated upon are lost to history, though Dr. Sims did mention three in his own writings: Anarcha, Betsey, and Lucy. In 2018, the statue standing in his honor in New York City's Bryant Park was removed, and the American College of Obstetricians and Gynecologists now each year recognizes February 28 through March 1, the days bridging Black History Month and Women's History Month, as the Betsy, Lucy, and Anarcha Days of Recognition. When we look back to Dr. Sims or laws that curtailed democracy, there is a tendency to place them safely in the past and presume them to be resolved problems. But violations of consent continued through the twentieth century, and the intertwining of law and medicine has now become even more tangled. Unconsented sterilization in California is still alleged as recently as the 2000s among imprisoned persons.[1] In many cases over the past decades, courts have also ruled that pregnant Jehovah's Witness patients could be transfused against their consent.

Over my career, I have managed many Jehovah's Witness patients. Like any group of people, they are not a uniform monolith but often heterogeneous in their beliefs, though collectively they will commonly decline blood transfusions. In 1985, a patient at eighteen weeks gestation was admitted to Jamaica Hospital in Queens, New York, bleeding from gastrointestinal varices. She refused blood transfusions on religious grounds, at which time the hospital urgently appealed to Judge Arthur Lonschein. Much of Judge Lonschein's subsequent written, formal opinion reads like a story written in prose, starting as follows:

> This past Saturday evening, April 20, 1985, at about 6:00 P.M., while I was getting dressed for a dinner engagement, I received a telephone call at my home from an attorney who identified himself as Mark Hartman, and who told me that he was associated with the firm of Hayt, Hayt Landau, Esqs.,

> representing Jamaica Hospital. He informed me that at the moment, the hospital had a patient suffering from internal bleeding and who was in critical condition. He further informed me that the patient was 18 weeks pregnant and had refused a blood transfusion necessary to stabilize her condition and to save the life of the unborn child.[2]

He goes on to describe personally entering the hospital with a tape recorder for a hearing on-site and being escorted by an officer into the patient's room in the ICU. Unlike other judges before and after who issued rulings from afar, he must have seen this patient directly, spoke to her, heard her pleas for bodily autonomy. He ruled against her and then walked out of the room, while the hospital proceeded to transfuse.

In 1996, Darlene Brown's physician scheduled the removal of a bladder polyp at Iglass Memorial Hospital in the southern suburbs of Chicago. She was thirty-four weeks pregnant at the time. The surgical plan was to anesthetize Brown with a spinal from the abdomen downward, then insert a scope into her bladder through which instruments could remove the polyp. In the operating room, she was anesthetized—numb, but otherwise remaining fully awake. The excision went awry, and Brown began bleeding profusely; the physician was unable to stop the hemorrhage, and her bladder was overflowing with blood. He called out from behind the sterile curtain for a blood transfusion, which was overheard by Brown herself, who in turn stated that she was a Jehovah's Witness. The physician had never before asked. It is interesting that court records describing this moment state, "Before the surgery, Brown did not discuss with Dr. Walsh that she was a Jehovah's Witness,"[3] the framing of which places responsibility squarely on the shoulders of Brown. An alternate phrasing could have been: "Before the surgery, Dr. Walsh did not ask Brown if she was a Jehovah's Witness." Regardless, the doctor now found himself starting into an uncontrolled, ongoing blood loss and a pregnant patient who did not consent to transfusion.

Finally, he was able to arrest the bleeding, after which Brown's hemoglobin plummeted to 3.4 g/dL—drastically, critically low, as normal hemoglobin in pregnancy is optimally at least three times higher at 11–12 g/dL. At 3.4, her heart and breathing raced as she struggled to maintain minimal blood pressure and oxygenation. At 3.4, it was amazing she was conscious or able to speak at all; at 3.4, many patients would have already died. Likely, Brown was about to die, as at a gestational age of thirty-four weeks she would inevitably deliver soon, with some additional blood loss certain even in uncomplicated deliveries and any additional loss fatal when already at 3.4. I do not presume to know Brown's own beliefs, though many individuals who are Jehovah's Witnesses believe that a transfusion precludes one from entering Heaven. What if these were also our beliefs? If faced with a choice between death on this earth and an eternity in Heaven, what would we choose?

On June 28, two days after the surgery, the State of Illinois filed a petition for adjudication of wardship and a motion for temporary custody of "Baby Doe," the fetus. Brown was unable to defend herself as she was hospitalized, barely alive, though her husband pled for her wishes to the bench. His arguments unheeded, the court instead appointed an administrator from Ingalls Memorial Hospital as the "temporary custodian of Fetus Brown, with the right to consent to one or more blood transfusions for Darlene Brown, when advised of such necessity by an attending physician."[4]

The hearing which had begun that morning concluded quickly by the same afternoon, and so that night the staff prepared to forcibly transfuse. In total, they infused six units of blood. I do not know why they chose six units specifically. Perhaps she still had ongoing bleeding that required additional transfusions, though presuming all bleeding had stopped, six full units would return someone to nearly normal versus only rescuing them from their immediate, life-threatening anemia. In addition, in a process that was certainly traumatic, an entire six units would need to transfuse over a long time. Likewise, we know that Brown's transfusions began on the evening of the 28th and did not conclude until the following afternoon, running hour by hour, drop by drop. What choices did she make over that time? Although details are scant, one fact is clear from legal records: Brown fought back. She "tried to resist the transfusions" and had to be "forcibly restrained, overpowered." The doctors were noted to have "yelled at" her and administered sedatives.[5]

When the staff walked into her room that night to transfuse, a bag of dark red blood in their hands, a court order against her placed in the chart,

Brown faced an inevitability; the doctors were determined, her immediate legal options were closed, and she herself was so anemic that she could likely barely move her arms, let alone wage physical defiance. But despite everything, she chose to fight that night. She fought despite being pregnant in the third trimester, despite a hemoglobin of 3.4 g/dL, despite having no hope at all. You can always choose to fight—even when fighting isn't logical, even when you cannot win. You can fight just because you believe something is wrong; you can fight because you simply want to fight, so that later you can tell yourself you fought. So, Brown fought.

Weeks later, she delivered her healthy child, and the legal case continued to move through the courts. Eventually, the Illinois Court of Appeals ruled that the transfusion had been improperly performed. Specifically, Brown should not have lost her right of refusal just because she was pregnant, as pregnancy did not negate basic bodily autonomy. This ruling has since remained a cornerstone of the legal arguments for pregnant Jehovah's Witness patients. I first learned about this story years ago from educational documents given to me by a patient. Brown remains the last known case of a competent, adult Jehovah's Witness patient in the United States transfused against their consent.

In medicine, the debate about patient consent is lively. At what reading level should a consent be written? Do we consider it consent when, at the end of commercials for a new drug, a narrator reads the laundry list of risks and side effects at comic speed? If a surgeon is describing to a patient their risks in a given operation, do they need disclose events with a probability of less than 1 percent, or are those sufficiently infrequent as to only frighten the patient or, worse, sway them against a surgery that is still of net benefit? What about risks that only occur in 0.1 percent of cases or 0.01 percent? What about risks that may exist but are currently unknown? Consent is far more complex than the patient just signing a piece of paper.

In law, the debate is ongoing as well. In 1978, the Court of the Central District of California heard the case of *Madrigal v. Quilligan*, in which ten Latina women alleged that they had been sterilized against their consent. It is noted that the defendant physicians maintain that proper consent was obtained and that all patients had understood and agreed to sterilization.

These assertions differ starkly from the sworn testimony of the women themselves, with aspects of the trial devolving into "he said / she said" types of debates. The stories from the ten women are all unique, and for some the defending hospital could not even produce a signed paper consent form, claiming over the women's vehement denials that they had agreed to sterilization verbally instead. For many plaintiffs, however, a recurring claim was that while they had signed their name to a paper consent form, it was in English, and they spoke Spanish. Thus, they had no concept of what they were told to sign, often just believing it to be consent for the cesarean itself, only later finding to their shock that they had been sterilized in violation of their desired family size. As presented in the documentary *No Mas Bebes*, many of these patients later mourned their lost fertility throughout their lives.

The counterarguments of the defending physicians included the simple fact that most patients had physically signed papers of consent. Thus, the technical criteria for consent had been fulfilled—an administrative standard that is comical, if not also tragic for these patients themselves. But there the consents were, submitted formally as exhibits at trial, physical pieces of paper emblazoned with the women's signatures, which could then be held in one's hands to examine. The judge, Jesse W. Curtis, ruled against the ten women in favor of the doctors and hospital.[6]

Consent is more than a singular action one makes with a pen: the patient signing a paper or a voter blackening an oval. Consent stretches through everything before and after those moments: the clarity of the explanations, the degree of understanding, and then, after the forms are signed or ballots cast, the actual translation of those decisions into actions. How does consent work in democracy? What information do voters receive as they head to polls, and who controls this information? What do we see on the physical ballots we hold in our hands? What then happens to our consent after election day ends?

Voters fundamentally support abortion rights, both overall and by even larger margins in cases of rape, incest, fetal anomalies, and endangered maternal health. Should the fundamental rights of some be electorally determined by the majority opinion of others in the first place? No. Certainly in the past, voters in many states, including Ohio, instead cast ballots to curtail the freedom of LGBTQ+ individuals to marry. Likewise, the language of reproductive amendments that would pass in a state are rarely those that would have been optimally preferred by the medical community. Leading up to the November 2023 election in Ohio, it was hard to not ponder an alternative in which others were voting upon my healthcare decisions instead. An individual's consent for their own care should be impervious to voters they will never meet. However, as the Dobbs ruling threw the issue of abortion back to the states, this is unfortunately the scenario in which we now find ourselves.

Ohio's reproductive freedom amendment, formally titled The Right to Reproductive Freedom with Protections for Health and Safety, was written to reflect the beliefs of our voters and pass. In an election for office, you may search for the ideal candidate, but ultimately that candidate is who they are, with all the blotches that humans may have. On election day, the candidate enters the booth with their flaws as their flaws, their skeletons in the closet as their skeletons. Alternatively, a ballot initiative is crafted from whole cloth; it can say exactly what you want it to say, do exactly what you want it to do. So you essentially write it to pass, construct it specifically to reflect the positions of over half the electorate—and our initiative was written as such, a mirror held up to the consent of the people. Thus, if all our voters simply rolled out of bed one morning, walked to their polling stations, read the amendment, and decided accordingly, it would pass without question. The amendment was also clear, with plain vocabulary, and short enough to be placed easily directly on a paper ballot and read in its entirety. The language thus was itself among our greatest assets, prepared diligently and thoughtfully over hours of meetings, with every individual word reflecting a decision. Certainly, our opponents knew this as well, which is why they went to such lengths to stop voters from seeing it in the booth. Thus, on election day, the language physically printed onto our paper ballots was amazingly not the actual words of the amendment for which we were voting; our legislators had used their power to place a thumb upon the scales of democracy.

Ohio law allows ballot boards to print a "summary" on the physical ballots rather than the unabridged, literal amendment itself. This is often reasonable, if not rational, as some amendments are interminably long or filled with legalese. This was the case for the same election's Issue 2, an initiative legalizing recreational marijuana, which was many pages long and thus impractical for unadulterated replication on paper. In these situations, the ballot board can either use a summary provided by the amendment's petitioners or craft a summary themselves so long as it remains honestly reflective. For example, the summary that appeared on paper ballots for recreational marijuana's Issue 2 was provided by the petitioners themselves.

For the reproductive freedom amendment, Issue 1, there was absolutely no need for a summary. We wrote it specifically to be read directly by voters: only 205 words in length and in plain English. The original "summary" concocted by our state leadership was in fact longer than the actual text it purported to summarize. They later shortened their final version to 193 words, but even then only rescued voters from an additional twelve words. The true reason was likely to not shorten or simplify the text, but to rather obscure voters, to unfairly sway them against it. The Ohio Secretary of State, to nobody's great surprise, explicitly stated after the election that he had written the "summary" in coordination with antiabortion groups.[7]

By way of example, consider the following actual wording of the amendment: "Abortion may be prohibited after fetal viability. But in no case may such an abortion be prohibited if in the professional judgment of the pregnant patient's treating physician it is necessary to protect the pregnant patient's life or health."[8] This was twisted on the voters' paper ballots into the following expression: "Always allow an unborn child to be aborted at any stage of pregnancy, regardless of viability if, in the treating physician's determination, the abortion is necessary to protect the pregnant woman's life or health."[9]

Among the many changes here was the replacement of "fetus" in the actual amendment with "unborn child" in the altered summary, removing the medically accurate expression with one overtly value-laden. In defending the choice, the Ohio attorney general's office asserted in a merit brief that voters might somehow not understand the word *fetus*, stating that "ballot language including the term 'fetus' has the potential to confuse voters, who may not know or understand the term's varying definitions."[10]

Was this legal? Our organization filed a lawsuit against the summary. In their counterarguments to our suit, abortion opponents asserted that their "summary" was not required to improve in any way the original language it was replacing, stating: "Over and over again, [the plaintiffs] insist that the amendment's text is better than the ballot language adopted by the Ballot Board, and because of this, the Ballot Board's chosen ballot language must be set aside in favor of the amendment's full text. But this Court does not decide whether other ballot language would have been better than the language ultimately adopted by the Ballot Board. The Court only decides whether the ballot language properly identifies the substance of the proposal to be voted upon and does not mislead, deceive or defraud the voters."[11]

In other words, it should not matter if it would actually be "better" to allow voters to see the true amendment so long as their summary was not misleading, defrauding, or deceitful. Our organization argued that the manipulated language was misleading and intended to defraud voters, though the Ohio Supreme Court, itself holding a majority of antiabortion justices, ruled predominantly against us, cementing the biased summary into the paper ballots.

As a physician and not a lawyer, I will defer questions of legality to others, though something certainly can be both legal and duplicitous. How does it constitute consent for voters if they cannot read on their ballots what they are actually voting upon? What if, as a physician, I changed my surgical consent in a manner similar to that in which our Secretary of State changed our ballots, replacing words and phrases prior to rolling the stretcher to the operating room? Voters, however, were not fooled by shenanigans, and Issue 1 passed by a margin of 57 percent to 43 percent. It went into effect thirty days after the election and is now written into our state's constitution.

I was incredibly nervous heading into that November election, pondering what would happen to myself and colleagues should it not pass, with us potentially then trapped for years in the horrible scenario that is right now faced by physicians in Texas, Tennessee, Idaho, and many other states. After it passed by such large margins, though, my prior anxiety felt almost silly. Abortion rights, after all, are popular in poll after poll, in state after state. But why then do these bans exist? In essence, they require our governors, legislators, and state attorney generals to act in opposition to the consent of the people, to actively labor against the will of the constituents one ostensibly serves. You can decide to impose abortion bans or uphold foundational beliefs of representative government, but not both.

Voters in North Carolina also support reproductive freedoms, and after the elections of 2022 they believed that their government would act in accordance with their consent. The supportive governor, Roy Cooper, had been elected earlier in 2020. Then in 2022, proponents successfully avoided a veto-proof majority of abortion opponents despite their legislative districts being grotesquely gerrymandered. In their house of representatives, however, the veto-proof majority was constrained by only a single seat. Among the legislators holding on tenaciously to abortion rights was a single representative from the 112th house district. She was a long-standing supporter of reproductive freedoms, as highlighted during a house debate in 2015 when she stated on the floor that, like many Americans, she had once had an abortion herself. In the wake of the Dobbs ruling, both abortion and LGBTQ+ rights were prominent in her election, a commanding 59 to 41 percent victory. Then through 2022 and early 2023, she likewise governed in concert with both her expressed opinions and the electorate's consent, including voting in 2023 in favor of an attempt to codify Roe into state law.

But in April 2023, to the shock of her constituents, the representative changed party affiliations.[12] On May 3, just months after she had voted to codify abortion rights, she cast the decisive vote for the veto override of a strict abortion ban. At the time of writing, North Carolina's ban remains in effect, impacting the lives of innumerable patients and healthcare workers, including inevitably many who had once cast ballots for the representative herself.

She was, of course, free to personally change her opinions, her views, or even her fundamental ideology, no matter how profound the metamorphosis. However, the decision to change your views and the decision to betray your electorate are two separate choices. There is no formal requirement that anyone remain a representative, such that if you determine that your new beliefs can no longer uphold the consent of those who placed you in office, then you can just step down rather than now cast votes against them.

Imagine a voter in the 112th house district who supports reproductive rights, voted for this representative specifically to secure those rights, and then find themselves personally in need of abortion but is now under a ban. Given the size of the district and the frequency with which people need abortion care, this scenario is unlikely to be hypothetical. In fact, the representative was once herself a voter in need of abortion. How many differing layers of consent—political, medical, democratic, bodily—would now be violated for this person, a virtual Russian doll of injustices?

What separates this representative from the physicians operating without consent as asserted by the plaintiffs in *Madrigal v. Quilligan*? She has never surgically touched a patient with her own hand, but she has altered medical care for hundreds of her electorate against their will: voters who did not sign a paper consent form but rather marked a dot on a ballot next to her name, never dreaming she would then do what she did. If you take either of these affairs and peel away all other professional, technical, legal, and administrative aspects until you are left only with the core of its consequence, each has begotten physical, real, medical subjugations of consent. The difference is just that one of the two acted only indirectly: their hands never needing sterile gloves, with them standing safely behind the legislative mechanizations of government.

What if physicians and legislators were held to the same standards of consent? What if upon entering a voting booth, the electorate was informed of the risks, benefits, and alternatives in a manner similar to that for medical interventions? What if after the election, our leaders were held to our consent like a surgeon caring for a now anesthetized patient? Election outcomes directly impact our health, so why is the bar set so much lower for democracy than medicine?

II MEDICINE BEFORE AND AFTER DOBBS

6 RUPTURE: PREVIABLE RUPTURE OF THE FETAL MEMBRANES

In December 2022, Anna Zargarian was seated with her bridesmaids on her wedding day, happily applying makeup, likely never imagining she would soon be a plaintiff against her state of Texas. As related first anonymously to NPR[1] then later under oath in a court of law, Zargarian, who was nineteen weeks pregnant at the time, suddenly experienced a gush of warm fluid. "It felt like something was coming out of me. So I freaked out. I literally wet my dress in the seat that I was in." She and her then-fiancé, now husband, Scott, left for the hospital, where they spent what had been planned as their wedding night in an emergency room instead, an impossible scenario now unfolding before them.

Membrane rupture, colloquially referred to as the "water breaking," occurs when the amniotic sac tears, allowing the fluid to exit through the cervix. It is usually depicted in movies and on TV as a dramatic event, with a pregnant character conversing over some plot detail when a rush of fluid precipitates the chaotic race to the hospital. Often, however, fluid leakage can occur subtly, sometimes as a slow trickle easily confused with vaginal discharge or loss of urine. Membranes rupture in a range of contexts and gestational ages. Most often they tear in response to uterine contractions in normal labor. Alternatively, membranes can be ruptured intentionally by a midwife or physician in concert with term induction. Sometimes, though, they rupture on their own prior to any symptoms or contractions—an unexpected surprise, as befell Zargarian.

When describing such a membrane rupture, the medical nomenclature is unfortunately idiosyncratic and often confusing. When *rupture of membranes* (ROM) occurs without uterine contractions prior to the onset of labor, it is referred to as *prelabor ROM* (PROM, pronounced phonetically like the formal dance at the end of high school). PROM can occur at any gestational age. When PROM occurs and the gestational age is also preterm, a second "P" is added to the abbreviation, which is then PPROM. In addition, PPROM will sometimes occur at a gestational age so premature that the fetus is not yet viable; that is, it could not yet survive if delivered. This was the unfortunate case for Zargarian, whose membranes ruptured at nineteen weeks and who thus had *previable PPROM*. The remainder of this chapter will likewise focus on previable membrane rupture, which will in turn just use the abbreviation PPROM for simplicity.

How does PPROM occur? Membranes can rupture from a direct physical injury to the uterus, such as a patient slipping on ice or being involved in a motor vehicle accident. However, this is uncommon as healthy amniotic membranes are actually quite strong, successfully holding in all the heavy fluid and uterine contents through weeks and weeks of normal pregnancies. In fact, membranes are often frustratingly intransigent to rupture when physicians are intentionally trying to do so. This is because they contain large quantities of collagen, the same molecule comprising your ligaments, tendons, and cartilage. When PPROM does occur, it therefore is often because enzymes—particularly a family of proteins called *matrix metalloproteinases* (MMPs)—have been activated and are degrading the membranes, causing them to weaken. Molecule by molecule, MMPs slice apart the collagen until they eventually render a tear. But why would the body activate these enzymes to cause rupture? Sometimes the reason is unknown, though often the body has identified either an infection or intrauterine bleeding, signaling a danger for the fetus and parent. Likewise, patients who experience PPROM without initial symptoms are often later found to be harboring intrauterine bacterial infections, initially silent absent the membrane rupture, which later cascade throughout the body into sepsis or even shock.

When a patient experiences PPROM in a restrictive state, what are the risks they face and what laws surround them? Since the Dobbs decision, PPROM cases have become a focus of intense debate, litigation, and human suffering, with tremendous variations from one state to the next.

Some abortion bans, such as in my state of Ohio, clearly listed PPROM as an exception. Thus, during the weeks of our law's enforcement, we continued to offer abortion for PPROM as we had done before. Many other bans, however, don't mention PPROM as either a specific exception or prohibition, leaving individual doctors or hospitals to decide if it instead falls under the affirmative defense as a threat to maternal health or life. Opinions in this regard varied widely, especially in the early days after Dobbs, creating situations in which one hospital in a given city would decide to not risk abortion for PPROM while a different hospital on another side of town may, with a patient's care varying depending upon which emergency room doors they walked through. Texas, for example, did not include guidance about PPROM in SB 8, resulting in many Texans being unable to access abortion. Later, in June 2024, Texas House Bill 3058 was passed, which provides a specific exception for PPROM—but not before innumerable patients had already been denied care and in many cases became profoundly ill.

In March 2022, with the Dobbs decision leaked but not yet formally released, another abortion ban, HB 598, was submitted to the Ohio legislature and then scheduled for testimony. HB 598 was somehow more extreme than our existing ban.[2] Specifically, it did not hold any exceptions for PPROM, such that, if passed, it would have thrown us and our patients into the situation faced by doctors in Texas at the time. Three Ohio physicians were thus set to testify against it—me and two colleagues in OB-GYN, one of whom was an infertility specialist as the new ban involved embryos as well. The prospect of live testimony made us nervous, especially the Q and A that would follow our prepared statements. Legislator questions are unpredictable and sometimes inflammatory, and the entire proceedings are recorded then made accessible forever online as public record. On the day before we testified, our team strategized answers to probable questions. I had a face sheet for the committee, from which we scrutinized the members themselves, mostly men smiling through bright white teeth and sharp suits. We outlined those who were supportive or not and which counterpoints could arise from whom. As we were finishing, I noticed that one of the legislators had not been discussed at all. "What about Representative X?" I asked.

Although this representative opposed abortion rights, they were also believed to be broadly disinterested, voting according to party but without passion; their legislative activities focused instead on taxes and bureaucratic restraint. There was no need to learn anything particular about them as the probability of a question from their direction was low.

The energy was palpable on the day of the hearing, occurring in that historic window between the leak and the release of the Dobbs decision. Our group of testifying physicians arrived early to enter the statehouse prior to protesters. At the start, the chair sounded the gavel and asked for decorum, and the session proceeded without hostility. I believe that day the legislators were listening, even if they did not agree; their questions were at least respectful and clearly given thought. This also proved the last hearing for that bill, which was shelved after our testimony, later dying in committee at the end of session. From the lectern, my colleagues and I surveyed the representatives, most of whom were engaged, looking forward, many taking notes. Then I glanced toward the back at the legislator who could not have feigned less interest. They looked down at their desk, then sometimes at us, then back down again, never raising a hand or uttering a word during the Q and A. And why would they? Their district was statistically antiabortion, so why would they ever logically evolve their position? They presumably did not believe the issue to be a personal concern. So why not just gaze away into space?

Of everyone in the chambers that day, I later wondered, who displayed the greatest raw power? The officer with badge and pistol guarding the door? The physicians at the lectern with years of experience? The chairman literally wielding a wooden gavel in their hand? Or the person with the power to not care about any of it at all?

In Ohio in 2022, a Hamilton County Common Pleas judge placed our state's entire ban under injunction, stopping all active enforcement and returning abortion to its prior legal status. A few weeks later, an MFM colleague of mine was consulted for a patient with previable membrane rupture. As is often the case, this patient initially had been in good health and experiencing a happy, uncomplicated pregnancy—until she called her general obstetrician because she was relentlessly leaking fluid. The obstetrician sent the patient to my colleague as the pregnancy was now high risk. After a compassionate, detailed, and likely painful conversation weighing risks and options, the patient decided it was best to discontinue the pregnancy, after which the MFM called the patient's generalist obstetrician to update them of the plan for abortion. The obstetrician then asked if the abortion was legal.

The question was utterly shocking, both because our ban was currently under injunction and thus unenforced and because even back when it was in place, PPROM had been a clear exception spelled out in the law. In other words, abortion for PPROM had never been illegal in our state. Confusion regarding the ban's nuances ran rampant outside of obstetrics—though for a physician in our own field, seeing pregnant patients in their office day in and day out, one would presume an understanding at least equivalent to that of a citizen regularly reading the newspaper. But like the state legislator in the committee hearing weeks before, why would this particular obstetrician actually need to follow our changing laws if they were personally uninterested? When complications arise that may require abortion, they transfer their patients to high-risk care.

For the patient counseled that day by my colleague, what are the options that exist after PPROM? Often there are no real choices to be made: When membranes rupture prior to viability, most individuals will deliver shortly thereafter, entering labor in the first twenty-four to forty-eight hours even if not contracting at the moment of rupture. In many cases, this is because bacteria are already present in the amniotic sac, triggering first the MMPs that physically weaken the membranes, then labor itself. However, in some, the uterine musculature remains initially quiet, with no infection initially present; the pregnancy may continue for weeks or even months, with the patient not delivering but also never resealing and fluid continuing to leak as the days elapse. Without the fluid in which the umbilical cord normally floats freely, a stillbirth from cord compression may occur. If a patient experiences neither labor nor stillbirth, then there exist significant medical risks to the patient themselves. Normally, amniotic membranes not only hold in the fluid but act as a barrier against vaginal bacteria ascending upward into the placenta. Thus, infections can later arise even if not initially present, and they can in turn escalate into sepsis, requiring, in the most severe cases, hysterectomy or ICU admission. Bleeding from a uterine wall detachment of the placenta, referred to as *abruption*, can likewise occur and also be catastrophic. The smaller number of patients who do continue without labor, stillbirth, infection, or bleeding are usually then hospitalized once they reach a gestational age at which neonatal intervention is possible, remaining hospitalized thereafter often for weeks until delivery.

Are there any good outcomes after previable PPROM, any patients on the outlying statistical tails who ultimately deliver in good health? Yes, there definitively are. Although most of my patients attempting continuation sadly did not succeed, I will always remember the small number who improbably remained free of additional complications and are the parents of a healthy child today. This fact makes previable PPROM more complicated than other scenarios in which healthy outcomes are impossible, such as unequivocally lethal anomalies.

For pregnancies that do progress, however, there also then exists the specter of pulmonary hypoplasia. Given that the uterus is filled with amniotic fluid, the circular tunnels of the fetal trachea, bronchi, and other airways of the lungs are also filled with fluid rather than air. The liquid coursing through the lungs' airways helps prop them open during early development, similar to one pouring water into a rubber glove, causing each finger to then stretch outward and downward from the liquid's mass. This pressure in turn supports the lung's ongoing growth and division into the appropriate number of branching airways. However, when membranes rupture, the amniotic fluid will exit the lungs as well, causing airways to deflate as if one cut a small hole in that water-filled glove, causing the fingers to collapse back upon themselves as the fluid drains. When this occurs later in pregnancy, such as when water breaks as a normal part of term labor, it is inconsequential; the deflating lungs are already mature and normally developed, about to refill with air upon the first breath. However, if rupture occurs very early, before the fetal airways have fully expanded and finished dividing into the required number of branches, then the lungs may not develop normally at all, a condition called *pulmonary hypoplasia*.

Sometimes we can diagnose pulmonary hypoplasia with certainty—for example, if there is a complete absence of fluid from the very beginning due to a fetal kidney anomaly. In previable membrane rupture, by contrast, the occurrence and severity of hypoplasia can be difficult to predict. Even our best ultrasounds are unable to see the pulmonary tree's detailed, small, individual branches. MRI for the diagnosis of pulmonary hypoplasia is promising but still in development. Thus some patients are given a guarded prognosis; their membranes rupture early, the fluid volumes are low, the probability of hypoplasia is high—but months later, to their joy, they deliver a screaming, bright-pink baby.

But sometimes instead there are patients for whom hypoplasia is possible, though less probable: patients with a prognosis that is good but not certain. As the first, then second day after rupture passes, they appear stable and appear to be in the fortunate minority without initial labor, stillbirth, infection, or bleeding. They nervously make it through the first week, then the second. Later, at an even more advanced gestation, they are admitted to the hospital, then stay with us for weeks on end. The fetal heart rate is monitored each morning; each day they are rounded on by our team. Over time, they accumulate hope, pick up crafts or new hobbies to pass the time, repetitively eat the hospital's food, are visited by volunteers with service animals. Sometimes they start a paint-by-numbers project, or perhaps a long book, then each morning on team rounds we see the painting progress or receive updates on the novel's plot. On the weekends, family and friends visit; sometimes their older children are desperately missing their parent. Then when the gestational age is sufficiently advanced, usually thirty-four weeks, we transfer them with excitement to labor and delivery, only then discovering hypoplasia. When a child is born with severe hypoplasia, they simply cannot breathe. The lungs are not functional; their chest will desperately rise and fall, never moving sufficient air. Then, after all the days in the hospital, all the cafeteria food, the paint-by-numbers work, the hours seated by the room's window reading a book, all the accumulated hope—everything sometimes then concludes in just minutes, sometimes just enough to wrap the child in a blanket to place into their parent's arms. Standing in the room on those days, you look back upon the preceding weeks, seeing now that hypoplasia had always been there, the dye always cast.

Many of these patients would never regret their decisions regardless of the final outcome, the time spent with the child after delivery meaningful even if far too short, the long hospitalization still worth the chance in the face of uncertainty. But a person has to freely choose to go down this road. Imagine the same sequence of events, but instead forced upon someone against their will by legislators. In many states right now across America, this is exactly what is occurring.

In Texas, the ban with no exception for PPROM, SB 8, went into effect in September 2021, before Dobbs itself. Researchers at the University of Texas Southwestern Medical Center (UT Southwestern) shortly thereafter began analyzing the outcomes of previable PPROM patients for whom abortion was newly illegal. In October 2022, they published their grim results in the *American Journal of Obstetrics & Gynecology*.[3] Twenty-eight patients had experienced previable PPROM without other initial complications and had then been forced by Texas to continue. For 25 percent of the patients, a portion of the umbilical cord or fetus itself, such as a small arm or leg, had actually prolapsed out through the now unprotected cervix and was lying in the vagina. Forced continuation in that context is wildly, illogically dangerous. Of the initial twenty-eight patients, 36 percent became infected, one of whom required admission to an ICU to save their life from sepsis. In addition, 18 percent of the patients required a blood transfusion from uterine bleeding, and the majority, 57 percent, experienced at least one or more adverse maternal events.

Of the twenty-eight patients forced to attempt pregnancy continuation, only eight fetuses were born alive; the other twenty fetuses were stillborn. Of those eight fetuses born alive, seven succumbed to extreme prematurity within just the first twenty-four hours. At the time the study was published, only one fetus from the original twenty-eight patients was alive, still hospitalized in the neonatal ICU with an unknown long-term prognosis or ultimate outcome.

On March 6, 2023, the Center for Reproductive Rights filed a lawsuit in Texas, *Zurawski v. State of Texas*, on behalf of two obstetricians and five patients denied abortion, expanded now to over twenty plaintiffs. Two of the original five patients had experienced PPROM, including the namesake Amanda Zurawski, whose membranes ruptured at eighteen weeks. Like the patients described in the UT Southwestern research, she was denied abortion under Texas law, then developed an infection that rapidly evolved into overwhelming sepsis, which she survived only after admission to the ICU.

Zargarian, whose membranes ruptured at nineteen weeks on her wedding day, is also now a plaintiff in that case. After consulting with physicians that night in the emergency room, she and her husband decided that rather than stay and await what may come, they needed to escape Texas to preserve her health. But how does a patient with PPROM actually, logistically, get out of a state? Beyond the sanitary question of relentlessly leaking amniotic fluid, a patient can bleed, enter labor, or deliver at any moment. When Anna purchased airline tickets to Colorado, she thus selected seats near the front so she could at least quickly run into the plane's small bathroom if needed. The flight was spent in a rational state of fear, wearing pads to collect the accumulating fluid while seated in her chair.

Ultimately, she made it safely to Colorado. Others throughout the country since Dobbs have not been as lucky. A practical question for those pregnant in states with bans to consider is how far away the nearest nonrestrictive state is. In an urgent situation, how would they get there? Where else in the country do they have friends, relatives, or support? What would their plan be for escape?

7 DISEASE: PREGNANCY WITH CONCURRENT MEDICAL ILLNESS

Among our most common patients in maternal fetal medicine are those pregnant with some other, unrelated, chronic health problem—for example, pregnant people with diabetes, liver disease, seizures, organ transplants, or thyroid conditions. When originally choosing which specialty to enter, this broad swath of medicine drew me into our field; rather than just focusing upon a single organ or system, I think constantly of the heart, the pancreas, or the brain. In hospital corridors, I talk with cardiologists, endocrinologists, urologists, and neurosurgeons. Likewise, training in MFM is broad, as we must learn from many different fields outside obstetrics itself.

When I was a resident, for example, I spent eight continuous weeks on the myocardial infarction service in cardiology. It was supposed to be a general medicine service and for only a few weeks, but when it came time for my rotation, the general unit was full with other residents from other fields, and so I was sent to cardiology instead. There, rather than being even in a broad cardiology service, I was placed on the specialized team managing *myocardial infarctions*—that is, heart attacks. During that month, one of my coresidents left the program. To adjust our schedules for the now-missing trainee, each block was lengthened by several weeks, including the cardiology rotation I was currently on. Thus, through a series of quirks, I came to spend eight long weeks as an obstetrics resident managing patients with heart attacks.

Eight weeks is far longer than most medical trainees rotate on a single service. During my eight weeks, other fellows, residents, and students would come and go, with me as the stable, consistent presence who knew the floor and patients. The senior cardiologists would cover seven days at a time—one physician working with me one week, then returning weeks later, confused to still see me. But after eight weeks you become an efficient, organized machine. The nurses came to know me, grabbing me in the hall when Mr. Smith had worsening chest pain. As the management of just myocardial infarction is narrower and more specialized, the initial steps were highly protocolized and well learned in the first week or two.

One night well into those eight weeks, an elderly man with chest pain was flown in by helicopter. I started through my steps, almost transcending the routine and into the prereflexive. I reviewed the history and EKG, examined the blood work, then called the senior cardiologist sleeping at home to formulate a plan for catheterization in the morning. Shortly thereafter the man's family arrived, delayed as they had traveled by car rather than helicopter. His wife was well-dressed despite the emergency and late hour, elderly but skilled in the art of graceful aging, and was flanked by her two adult sons. All three had the sorts of expressions seen in situations both urgent and deep in the night: a combination of fatigue, alarm, and determined focus. I led them down the hall to the family conference room, windowless, though with some milquetoast pastoral painting and a continuously replenished box of tissues. I explained everything with authoritative reassurance, employing the communication skills I first learned in medical school. Her husband had likely suffered a myocardial infarction, or heart attack, but he was currently stable and receiving all appropriate medications. I explained that in a few hours he would undergo cardiac catheterization, with the catheter to be inserted through a large vein. We would know more after that, though many patients suffer heart attacks and then recover in adequate health. He was in competent hands. While I was talking, his wife remained nervous, though perhaps now more centered. Finished, I asked gently if they had questions, which was when I first noticed the son sitting to his mother's right. Concerned, he was staring straight at my white coat—specifically, the space above my left pocket where my specialty's name was embroidered in thick black thread—and yes, he definitely had a question: "Are you . . . an obstetrician?"

"Yes," I said, truthfully though awkwardly, my performative expertise a sudden simulacrum. But as out of place I may have been that night in cardiology, why do cardiologists in training not alternatively rotate through obstetrics? Or endocrinologists, nephrologists, or psychiatrists? Just as obstetricians still need to know about the heart, every medical specialty caring for reproductive-age patients must know about pregnancy, because everyone in clinical medicine will see pregnant people. They will come into the ER after car accidents, be psychiatrically hospitalized, or be rolled into operating rooms with appendicitis. The cardiologist needs to know how pregnancy impacts the heart; the nephrologist, the kidney.

Likewise, all doctors need to know about abortion. Right now, statewide bans vary enormously in their guidance and exceptions for medical conditions. If a person is considering pregnancy in a restrictive state and has a chronic health condition, they should investigate the abortion laws specific to them. Talk to specialists about your plans for pregnancy ahead of conception to ensure you both are currently optimized and have a plan for if the disease worsens while pregnant. In fact, even if you are completely healthy, it is prudent to see your primary care physician in the year prior to conception to ensure you are up to date with screening studies, adult vaccinations, and other preventative measures. MFM physicians are also available for preconception consultations. Although we do not actively manage individuals who are not pregnant, and generally our offices are only filled with obstetric patients, we happily see people who are not yet pregnant but have health conditions in order to construct a future plan. We review records to ensure they are optimized and review medications to see which would be safely continued or discontinued upon conceiving. We describe what a pregnancy would be like, what risks their disease would entail.

The mirror image of such planning is the patient in poor health who suddenly, unexpectedly, finds themselves pregnant with their disease uncontrolled, their medications teratogenic. This situation is always best avoided, but now more so in states under bans. The responsibility for preventing this scenario likewise falls upon every physician, not just those of us in obstetrics—and prevention is quite straightforward. The American College of Obstetricians and Gynecologists recommends that once a year every patient capable of pregnancy be asked a simple question: "Would you like to become pregnant in the next year?"[1] This question does not have to be asked by an ob-gyn; it can be raised by a primary care physician or even a pediatrician. It can be asked by a cardiologist to a patient with heart disease, an endocrinologist to a patient with diabetes, a rheumatologist to a patient with lupus—but someone needs to ask this short question once a year. If the answer is no, then explore the need for contraception, referring to gynecology if the physician is not themselves comfortable in this arena. If the answer is yes and the patient is medically complicated, send them to MFM. For so many patients right now in so many states that have abortion bans, this one simple question is our primary weapon against endangerment.

In the aftermath of Dobbs, I fielded nervous questions about such patients from physicians in anesthesiology, emergency medicine, radiology, pharmacology, and other fields, doctors who had perhaps once believed that abortion bans did not impact them, that perhaps they were separated from obstetrics by magical shields. Then one day after the bans, a radiologist worries about fetal X-ray exposure, an anesthesiologist about anesthetics; a cardiologist agonizes over a pregnant patient with heart disease descending into failure, their lungs flooding with fluid. MFM specialists are never alone in our boats. If I have a pregnant patient with cancer, for example, I am finding an oncologist and bringing them onto this boat with me. They may not want to be on this boat, perhaps disliked the boat back in medical school, may find these waters frightening—but here we are.

Patients newly diagnosed with cancer usually assume abortion to be an inevitability, believing pregnancy and cancer to be incompatible. Sometimes this is entirely true, such as when therapies inconsistent with pregnancy must be urgently deployed against aggressive malignancies. But many are surprised to instead discover a nuanced landscape with continuation a potential path, albeit one still fraught with risk—risk that must be understood, accepted, and then chosen freely. For example, a tumor in a location distant from the pelvis, such as a limb, can be surgically removed without direct fetal risks. A surprising number of chemotherapeutics are well studied in pregnancy with acceptable obstetric outcomes. Every cancer story is unique, resisting one-size-fits-all recommendations. Even in pregnancy, and even regarding abortion.

I once counseled a patient recently diagnosed with cancer in the first trimester. A small mass had been found, sampled with a thin needle, and then evaluated under the microscope; the pathologist viewed a slide covered in malignancy. The patient now sat in my office bravely projecting stoicism, presuming abortion to be my recommendation. However, I counseled that this was not actually straightforward. Although cancer was firmly diagnosed, we did not yet know the *stage*—that is, how far through the body malignant cells may or may not have spread. Seen on imaging so far was only the solitary mass, with her other organs reassuring in appearance. Thus, it was possible she was in stage I, the cancer confined to a single location, resolvable after surgical excision. Her mass also resided outside the pelvis, presenting a negligible physical risk to the pregnancy itself. Of course, it may not be stage I; the spread of cancer could potentially be present, just not yet seen. The next step was for surgical removal, followed by the pathologist carefully reviewing the slides, millimeter by millimeter, to determine if all visible cancer had or had not been completely excised. If ultimately the cancer was stage I, then no other treatments would be required during pregnancy, which could just proceed normally. For years to follow, she would undergo surveillance to guard against recurrence, though this would all be after the delivery. In addition, if it was stage II or greater, requiring chemotherapy, there still existed treatments for this specific cancer that were employable in pregnancy. Thus, from our current vantage point, I did not see an absolute recommendation for abortion. I told her she could, if desired, continue, pending the results from pathology.

But continuation would still be a strain in even the best scenario. Although surgery could be safely performed, she would have to simultaneously endure postoperative recovery and pregnancy, a wearing endeavor to which my wife could attest, having undergone emergency surgery mid-pregnancy herself for an ovarian mass. For any abdominal surgery, the scar then stretches from the expanding uterus over the next weeks while trying to heal. The cancer also easily could require chemotherapy, which is often harrowing even when a patient is not also pregnant. Envision the common chemotherapy side effects—nausea, fatigue, mental cloudiness—and then the usual symptoms of pregnancy, then both combined at the same time. Finally, even if the surgery was successful, the cancer was stage I, and the pregnancy proceeded normally, her future would still hold an ongoing risk of recurrence. What if, one or two years later, metastases emerged that required more surgery and chemotherapy, which she would now face while also managing a small child?

I must note here that this case was many years in the past, long before the Dobbs decision. Like hundreds of examples across the entire array of human diseases, how would any physician now know how to manage this case under restrictive bans?

But that day, long before Dobbs, we reviewed everything in detail. Ultimately, the patient revealed that her feelings toward the pregnancy had actually been ambiguous, an ambiguity independent of and predating the discovery of her cancer. She was uncertain if this was the best time for another child given her finances, stresses, and other children and had been considering abortion even before the diagnosis. As soon as she said this, I realized my mistake in first lunging into a long conversation about surgery and chemotherapy before asking if she even wanted to be pregnant in the first place.

In my subspecialty, I can risk myopically focusing on only the most complicated aspects of a case without first seeing the overall picture. I often need to remember that most obstetric patients never need to talk to me, as they freely enjoy their healthy pregnancies. Likewise, the healthy patients for whom abortion is simply their best choice are usually not my patients as I see only complicated patients and circumstances. But it is difficult to retain your view of normal while all day long seeing convolutions. For example, pediatric cancer is also statistically rare, but when my wife looks out into the world, she often sees cancer everywhere as well. Any semblance of actual numerators and denominators were long ago smashed with hammers for both of us.

My skewed perspective can be problematic when publicly advocating for reproductive rights, as focusing on my patients with medical complications is at best statistically nonrepresentative or worse insinuates a hierarchy of deservedness, dividing those seeking abortion into "bad" or "good" groups in accordance with their circumstance. Patients seeking abortion never need justify their decisions to others, let alone have cancer or even cancer of a given stage. Ultimately, the patient that day chose abortion followed by the surgical removal of the tumor, which then microscopically appeared entirely contained. No chemotherapy was needed; her future only held recurrence monitoring after surgical recovery.

Years later, I strolled into our office, the waiting room of which was shared with the general clinic. On my way in, I saw a pregnant woman I recognized but did not immediately place in my memory. I settled into my desk with the patient bouncing about my head until I suddenly recalled her as the cancer patient from years before, now pregnant again and apparently free from recurrence. This sequence of events is common for patients who choose abortion: As evidenced in the Turnaway Study[2] and elsewhere, many patients who seek abortion later still welcome children under more optimal circumstances. I reflected on how relaxed the patient appeared relative to our visit years before, now following in the general practice and no longer needing a high-risk specialist such as me.

After logging in and checking the day's schedule, I meandered to the workroom, where the resident assigned to the patient was seated in front of her computer. I told her I was happy to have seen my former patient in the waiting room looking cheerful and well.

"Yes," the resident replied with a smile, "she's particularly grateful after an abortion had been required the last time."

"What are you talking about?" I asked, smiling less.

The patient, the resident explained, described her prior pregnancy as unplanned but desired. She had wanted to continue but was told, by me, that abortion was an unavoidable necessity, with pregnancy in the context of cancer impossible. She thus proceeded regretfully, the procedure not her decision.

This was not remotely truthful. Our conversation years before had been extensive and nuanced, options of both continuation and discontinuation explored in detail, her decision made freely. Why was she now spinning the resident a falsehood? Perhaps a story in which she was given no choice was easier than one where she faced entangled options. Perhaps this was only a small lie. She did, after all, truly have cancer, and abortion in this context was entirely reasonable. Certainly, if an acquaintance asked about the abortion she could just say "cancer," without needing additional details. But the lie involved me, casting me in a dictative light, if not even ominous, and with my described advice also medically incorrect. In addition, the story fundamentally framed abortion as needing medical justification, unacceptable if it was only a person's own best choice. In this story, hers had been a "good" abortion rather than one of the "bad" ones.

The patient was now checked in awaiting her visit, the room number visible on the resident's screen. I strode down the hall and opened the door; the patient sat in the chair fully dressed. She first smiled warmly in recognition, though with a hint of worry in her face, realizing perhaps her prior mistruths.

"You told the resident I had said abortion was required, that it was unavoidable despite you not wanting one," I said, "that I told you there was no choice. You know that is not true. Your decision was reasonable, had my support, but was a choice."

She did not reply but rather sat quietly, with me becoming aware of my actions like someone gazing suddenly into a scene rather than just being an actor within it. The scene I now saw was utterly unprofessional. The irony was that I chastised her for having had a choice, though at that moment she would have certainly chosen to not have me there standing over her. After uncomfortable seconds, I meekly wished her well and stepped out. I circumvented the workroom as I returned to my office; in my embarrassment, I did not want to see the resident.

If the patient decided to change her story, to even outright lie, to even lie about me, that was her choice to do so; we are her physicians and not her moral arbitrators. If a doctor must choose between fairness and care, we choose care. The patient that day drove to her doctor's office for care, not to a lawyer's office for examination or a clergyman for absolution. Although we carry everywhere our own moral compass, we do not sit upon thrones from which to adjudicate patients' choices.

Physicians require empathy for the decisions our patients make and experiences we may not understand. I have never had cancer and will never be pregnant, let alone be pregnant with cancer, but I have to empathize despite experiencing neither. There is, after all, no broad expectation that doctors have the experiences of our patients. My wife has a small number of colleagues who are themselves survivors of childhood cancer. However, such individuals are quite uncommon, with the predominance of pediatric oncologists having never taken their patients' harrowing journeys. All gerontologists, unless they work long into later life, will never in their career experience being elderly. There exist many exceptional pediatricians who, either by choice or circumstance, have never themselves been parents, and despite that they spend enriching careers skillfully counseling on teething, toilet training, and temper tantrums. Theodor Geisel, better known by his pen name, Dr. Seuss, authored imaginative, groundbreaking books for children while having never had children himself, famously stating, "You make 'em, I amuse 'em."[3]

Although we do not require our own experiences, we do require empathy to the experiences of others. Sadly, we do not always achieve this goal, especially for patients who may differ demographically from us. Unacceptable racial disparities exist in the United States for essentially all obstetric outcomes, including maternal and infant mortality. The causes are multifactorial, but they certainly include systemic racism, which can manifest as physicians not believing the experiences reported to them by their patients. Concerns and symptoms are then often dismissed. In a 2021 linguistic analysis of medical records, physicians were significantly more likely to sew doubt into information presented by Black patients, disproportionally using words such as *claims* or *insists* rather than just accepting facts at face value.[4] The institution of medicine as a whole has also long ignored or minimized the complaints of female patients.

What of the legislators writing abortion bans? The legislators surveying the universe of different human diseases and then deciding which conditions will or will not receive exceptions? What medical phenomena may they have also experienced? When Ohio's ban was written in 2019, there was likely at least one legislator with some personal understanding of reproductive decisions in the context of medical illness. I do not know who it was, or their exact story, but when you read the law's text you can see the clue left behind, a small puzzle piece that doesn't fit but clearly was added by someone with the political power to do so. The bill listed only five exceptions, with all other abortions for maternal health relegated to affirmative defense. During the months of the ban's enforcement, doctors memorized those five crucial exceptions: (1) preterm premature rupture of membranes, (2) preeclampsia,

(3) diabetes, (4) vaginal bleeding, and (5) multiple sclerosis (MS). Of the five, MS stands out unequivocally from the others.

MS is a rare disease, affecting less than 0.5 percent of the population. Despite this, I have cared for many pregnant MS patients as it affects females more often than males, and the mean age of diagnosis is the late twenties to early thirties, overlapping with the age when most pregnancies also occur. The cause of MS remains frustratingly unclear, but it ultimately results in inflammatory attacks upon myelin, the protective coat overlying the portions of nerve cells that conduct electric signals to our body. If the long portion of a nerve, called the *axon*, is thought of as a metal wire, then myelin would be the plastic protective sheath. MS specifically impacts the central nervous system, including the brain and spinal column. Because it affects so many different types of nerves, the disease can manifest in a wide array of symptoms. Pain is common and can strike anywhere in the body. Patients may have loss of sensation or weakness in their limbs or urinary or fecal incontinence from the nerves controlling the bladder or bowel. Visual disturbances may arise from the eye's optic nerve. Finally, MS can manifest in the brain itself: fatigue, depression, cognitive impairment, and seizures.

Pregnancy with MS can likewise be arduous. If MS impacts a person's legs, then trips and falls with resultant uterine injury become a constant risk. After delivery, MS flares may increase due to immunologic alterations and the sleep deprivation that accompanies infant care. As anyone with a newborn knows, the first weeks after delivery can be rough under even the healthiest circumstances. How would a person manage symptomatic MS while also staying up all night with diaper changes and feeding?

However, from the standpoint only of quantifiable obstetric risks, the great majority of pregnancies in patients with MS result in healthy deliveries to parents whose disease then continues unchanged. For MS patients, having or not having a child does not appear to alter their long-term disease trajectory. Although MS may worsen for a while after delivery, the rate of relapse for stable patients will actually decrease during the pregnancy itself. The relationship likely works both ways in that MS also does not appear to impact pregnancy risks. Compared to healthy individuals, patients with MS are not found to suffer increased rates of birth defects, miscarriage, preterm birth, or stillbirth. Most patients I have cared for with MS have enjoyed uncomplicated term deliveries.

None of which should suggest that MS patients should not have access to the full range of reproductive choices or that abortion may not be the best option for an individual person with MS. Certainly, if I had a patient with MS who desired abortion, they would have my support, and apparently the support of our legislators writing the state law in 2019 as well.

So of all the hundreds if not thousands of human diseases, with only five named exceptions, why did our leaders specifically select MS? Fundamentally, I do not know. I was not there, as nobody crafting the legislation sought either my opinion or that of the American College of Obstetricians and Gynecologists, the Society for Maternal-Fetal Medicine, or any equivalent professional organizations. But someone had to have made the decision to select MS, someone in a position of power. The five exceptions were not selected randomly by a legislator throwing darts at a medical textbook. It is impossible not to speculate on the decision coming from a place of personal experience, as MS is otherwise too idiosyncratic a selection.

Sometimes our lived experience expands our view of the world, our empathy. For some people, however, a lived experience may close doors rather than open them. A person may believe that their own experience is now valid above others, not having the imagination to consider otherwise. In 2019, before introducing their abortion ban, legislators presumably had one or maybe many meetings to craft the ban's specific language, with the group debating under which scenarios abortion was, in their own opinions, acceptable—essentially, which patients would have rights and which would not. No exception was made for rape. No exception was made for incest. But someone clearly requested an exception for MS. What was their justification? Did they have a loved one suffering from MS? Had a family friend with MS chosen abortion? Maybe they had MS themselves and could not imagine the strain of a pregnancy? Whatever the answer, it was likely was an understanding of this disease as a lived experience. However, it also constituted the limit to which they imagined or cared. Whatever their experience was, they used their power to create a literal exception for the disease they knew, MS—but only MS and four others.

8 TORCH: TRANSPLACENTAL FETAL INFECTIONS

Fortunately, most maternal viruses and bacteria do not also infect the fetus. Protection against pathogens is one of the placenta's many jobs, and placentas are arguably the most fascinating of all organs. They diffuse oxygen and CO_2, like our lungs; electrolytes, like our kidneys; nutrients, like the gastrointestinal track; and synthesize a wider array of hormones than any other endocrine organ—all while also erecting barriers against agents harmful to the fetus.

But no defense is always immutable. A small number of pathogens can still cross into the uterine cavity and sometimes inflict terrible damage there. In medical school, students learn the acronym *TORCH* to memorize the most common infections that risk fetal injury. Classically, TORCH stands for *toxoplasmosis, rubella, cytomegalovirus, and herpes*. The acronym is flawed in part because it does not include new, harmful viruses we identify over time—most recently, Zika. It also importantly excludes syphilis. However, as medical shorthand, pathogens capable of fetal injury are collectively called *TORCH infections*.

The outcomes from TORCH vary, from completely asymptomatic newborns to tragic neurologic devastation and everything in between. Cytomegalovirus (CMV), for example, is the most common cause of nongenetic congenital hearing loss. Toxoplasmosis infections risk visual impairment. As a result, patients will sometime choose abortion in cases of early and severe infections. However, most state abortion laws contain no mentions of TORCH. Ohio's ban prohibited any abortion for fetal indications, which would presumably include TORCH infections. Louisiana's list of life-limiting fetal conditions also did not include TORCH.

Understanding how to avoid infections and what to do if one occurs is important for all prenatal patients regardless of location, though it is also now more urgent under abortion bans without fetal exceptions. So what are these infections, how does the body's immune system fight against them, and what should a person do in cases of exposure?

If I were an immunologist researching our body's intricate networks of antibodies, white blood cells, and cytokines, I would find pregnancy fascinating. In pregnancy, our immune system must evolve to accommodate the fetus, which is genetically and thus immunologically dissimilar to the parent. The mechanism remains unclear, though a gross oversimplification is that immunity dials back a bit in pregnancy. Thus, diseases in which our immune systems are the culprits—autoimmune and inflammatory conditions such as lupus, Crohn's disease, or MS—often improve. The trade-off, however, is vulnerability to infections. If two people contract the flu, with one pregnant and the other not, the pregnant patient faces greater risks of hospitalization, intubation, and even death. Varicella, better known as chickenpox, is overtly dangerous in pregnant adults but usually mild in children. Obstetric patients are more prone to bladder infections, which can then spread to the kidneys, with kidney infections in turn precipitating sepsis and shock. Likewise, pregnant people proved especially vulnerable to COVID-19, and in 2020 the virus ripped mercilessly through our population. Progressively in Cleveland, we had our first pregnant patient, then our second, then numerous throughout our floor struggling to breathe on cannulas and face masks. Grief counselors after stillbirth traditionally collect ink handprints from the fetus for parents to always remember. During COVID, some instead collected, for surviving infants, the ink handprints of their dying parents.

One of the pandemic's early questions was if pregnant individuals should be formally considered immunosuppressed. Classic immunosuppressed patients are those with weakened immune systems from cancer, chemotherapy, or diseases such as HIV. In 2020, many hospital protocols divided patients or employees into binary categories of being or not being immunosuppressed for purposes of additional protection or access to treatments.

Pregnant patients have altered immunity, but were they then formally immunosuppressed? And if so, then should pregnant healthcare workers stay home rather than risk exposure from their patients?

During my wife's pregnancies, she would sometimes find herself managing cancer patients who were ill from TORCH pathogens while herself vulnerable. Years ago, early in our third pregnancy, she cared for a hospitalized child who was ill. Though initially undiagnosed, the child was later found to be infected with CMV, the *C* in *TORCH*. Fortunately, the risk of healthcare workers contracting CMV from clinical exposures is profoundly small, as transmission requires close contact with bodily fluids such as saliva or urine. Standard employee protections against infection, such as masking and gloves when required or scrupulous hand hygiene, are also usually sufficient to prevent TORCH. As a result, CMV testing is not recommended after a workplace exposure so long as the pregnant patient is otherwise asymptomatic. Instead, our primary risks of TORCH occur not from our work but from the wider world that exists after we walk out of the hospital doors.

For example, eating raw or undercooked seafoods or meats, unwashed produce, or unpasteurized milk and cheeses risks pathogens. *Listeria monocytogenes* is a bacteria capable of crossing the placenta and causing stillbirth, as well as often a source of national food recalls ranging from luncheon meats to cantaloupe to yogurt. Whenever a recall is announced, appropriately nervous patients who may have eaten the food in question frequently call obstetric offices. Fortunately, the risks are low after a recalled ingestion so long as the patient remains asymptomatic. If, however, a person has consumed a recalled product and then feels unwell—experiencing fever, nausea, loose stools, muscle aches—then a workup for listeria should be initiated.[1]

Toxoplasmosis, the *T* in *TORCH*, is also contracted by eating raw or undercooked meat, though unlike listeria it is more ubiquitous and sporadic rather than being a common focus of national recalls of specific foods by specific vendors. *Toxoplasma gondii* is a protozoan parasite with a complicated life cycle centered around felines—in particular, our common housecats. Infected felines excrete toxoplasmosis in their stools, prompting the classic recommendation that pregnant people not change litter boxes. However, the risk from a domestic cat is low presuming proper precautions, especially as cats only contract toxoplasmosis from eating raw meat. Thus, a strictly indoor cat should, in theory, not be at risk if it is eating only kibble. Cats that are infected, however, may defecate outside, making toxoplasmosis broadly present in soil, the plants that grow in soil, and the meat of animals that eat those plants. In addition to litter boxes, then, pregnant patients should also wear gloves when gardening, wash fruits and vegetables, and thoroughly cook meats.

When they do occur, obstetric infections with toxoplasmosis can be devastating. The parasite can embed within the fetal eyes, brain, liver, and spleen. Ultrasound findings can include enlargement of the liver or spleen, with bright areas in the fetal abdomen implying infection of the gastrointestinal track and structural injury to the brain. However, a predominance of infected newborns also ultimately deliver in good health, and antibiotics against toxoplasmosis exist. Decision-making in fetal cases therefore is quite complicated—and now all the more so in states with abortion bans.

One of the other most common fetal infections, syphilis, is of course avoided by strategies more complicated than washing fruits or thoroughly cooking steaks. Syphilis can cross the placenta and, similar to toxoplasmosis, infect the fetal brain, liver, eyes, and other organs. Bone marrow infections can cause profound fetal anemia. Syphilis also burrows into the fetal bones and teeth, producing lasting damage. Children born with syphilitic bones risk fracture throughout their lives. Teeth are classically deformed as well, given names such as *Hutchinson's teeth*, which are notched in the center, and *mulberry molars*.

Many of the TORCH infections either lack any treatments or only have therapies that are complicated, if not experimental. Toxoplasmosis, for example, often requires a special antibiotic imported from Canada or France as it is commercially unavailable in the United States. Syphilis, by contrast, is treated in pregnancy with penicillin—just normal, boring penicillin, the same antibiotic we have had for decades upon decades. Thus, in any optimal healthcare system, the number of babies born each year with congenital syphilis should be zero. Likewise, when I was a medical student, syphilis was profoundly rare, taught about in classrooms as if it was a historical disease from the past. In many ways, it was; I was several years removed from training before I ever saw my first case. Now, however, we see syphilitic patients constantly as it has exploded in concert with our national failure of public health. The number of babies born each year in the United States with syphilis, a number which should be zero, has increased 755 percent between 2012 and 2021.[2] As a result, the American College of Obstetricians and Gynecologists released an updated Practice Bulletin in 2024,[3] recommending that all pregnant patients, regardless of demographics or perceived risk factors, be tested for syphilis three times: at the beginning, in the second trimester, and upon arrival at the hospital for delivery.

But among all the TORCH infections, the most common remains CMV. According to the American College of Obstetricians and Gynecologists,[4] CMV infects between 0.7 and 4 percent of all pregnant patients. Because not all maternal infections cross the placenta, the rate of subsequent neonatal infections is 0.2 to 2.2 percent. Although probabilistically uncommon in an individual pregnancy, when extrapolated over the millions of births each year this incidence equates to thousands upon thousands of neonates, making CMV the most common infection—outpacing toxoplasmosis, listeria, and all others. CMV is a member of the Herpesviridae family of viruses, though otherwise quite dissimilar to its cousin, herpes simplex. Rather than soil, cats, or undercooked meats, it is transmitted from human to human via secretions such as saliva and urine. Infections in adults are generally mild so long as the adults are not immunosuppressed. If I had CMV right now, it may only feel like a mild, common cold; or, being fully immunocompetent, I may easily have no symptoms at all. For immunosuppressed patients, however, CMV can cause life-threatening infections of the lung, liver, or other organs. Thus the virus commonly haunts patients in cancer units, including the children cared for by my wife.

A few days after caring for her CMV patient, my wife experienced symptoms of a mild cold—perhaps unrelated, though she obtained blood work as a precaution. We were not initially worried as many healthcare workers already have immunity from prior exposures, but the labs demonstrated not only vulnerability but evidence of a recent new infection. It was confirmed a week later through specialized antibody assays, with our concern now escalating.

What is the management of a pregnant patient who has contracted CMV? Especially if that patient is now living in a state with restrictive laws? Toxoplasmosis can be treated with antibiotics, syphilis with simple penicillin. At the time, several years ago, the question we faced was whether to administer *CMV hyperimmune globulin*, an infusion of pooled targeted antibodies. The rationale for the infusions was straightforward: These are antibodies aimed specifically against CMV, not only fighting the parental infection but crossing the placenta to hopefully prevent or treat fetal infections as well. In 2005, researchers published a paper in the prestigious *New England Journal of Medicine* in which hyperimmune globulin was administered to pregnant participants newly infected with CMV like my wife.[5] The infusions appeared dramatically, almost miraculously, effective, reducing transplacental viral passage and improving fetal outcomes. Thus, use was spreading in Europe, with the medication also available in the United States but not formally approved in pregnancy by the FDA.

Although the results of the study were dramatic, it was also not a randomized trial; participants receiving infusions had self-selected rather than being assigned randomly with others receiving a placebo instead. Randomized trials are the gold standard for medication efficacy as outcomes can otherwise be highly confounded. Specifically, patients who actively seek then successfully receive experimental treatments differ meaningfully from those who do not, being often wealthier or benefiting from higher degrees of education, medical literacy, or personal connections within medicine. These factors may then, in an illusion of beneficence, account for the perception of improved outcomes rather than the novel treatment itself.

Evaluating outcomes after CMV infection is complicated further by the fact that most patients will do well even without treatment. Most maternal infections do not actually cross the placenta, and even then most fetal infections do not result in permanent harm; our immune systems usually fight the virus into retreat unassisted. Thus, despite the fanfare surrounding the published study, it remained possible that the results would have been the same without hyperimmune globulin, with apparent improvements attributable only to nonrandom selection.

Of course, it was also possible that hyperimmune globulin was perfectly effective as it consisted, after all, of concentrated CMV-specific antibodies. Randomized trial or no randomized trial, how could it even be logical that these antibodies would not help patients such as my wife? In addition, although someone's own immune system will successfully defeat most infections, the alternative of fetal injury was terrifying. Fetal neurologic infections can range from mild impairment to deafness to widespread outright destruction of brain matter.

Thus the question at that time facing not just my wife and I but the entire field of obstetrics was how to clinically approach the use of hyperimmune globulin. Broadly, there were two groups, one of which believed the infusions should be adopted immediately and routinely: The plausibility of benefit was too great, the nonrandomized data too compelling, the neurologic injuries too tragic to await years of additional study rather than act now with the research at hand.

To this day, neither my wife nor I belong to that broad ideological camp; we are aligned instead with those who support large-scale randomized trials ahead of routine clinical implementation, the camp referred to loosely if not always precisely as supporting *evidence-based medicine*. The history of medicine is replete with interventions prematurely adopted based on mechanistic plausibility, theories, or patient experience prior to actual clinical trials. These interventions are then later proven over and over again to be useless or even harmful.

At the time of my wife's infection, the National Institutes of Health's Maternal Fetal Medicine Units (MFMU) was, in fact, undertaking a large randomized trial of hyperimmune globulin for pregnant patients with CMV. Complicating matters for us, though, was that it was ongoing in only the handful of participating MFMU centers, the nearest of which was several hours away, making enrollment impractical. However, a patient could still potentially receive hyperimmune globulin outside of the trial as a physician could just order the infusion in a straightforward manner; the antibodies were commercially available even if not specifically approved for pregnancy. For colleagues such as myself who supported the trial, though, such off-label infusions were discouraged. Part of the reason entailed consistency in research ethics; that is, if hyperimmune globulin was considered experimental, then administration should only happen through the auspice of a trial under review board oversight. This would in turn be inconsistent with routine use even at other institutions not under the same board. The other concern was practical in that widespread nonexperimental use would simply erode enrollment in the trial, potentially even precipitating study failure. Thus, as an adherent to this ideological camp, I discouraged hyperimmune globulin at my institution prior to my own wife's infection. The pregnant patients whom I would see infected or exposed to CMV often specifically would be my fellow healthcare workers, medically educated and arriving in my office having read the *New England Journal of Medicine* study and terrified of fetal neurologic damage. I would then recommend that hyperimmune globulin remain only investigational; the subsequent conversations were often uncomfortable.

So ultimately, we decided to forgo the infusions ourselves, with the next step instead a series of ultrasounds to evaluate for any markers of fetal infection. Weeks later, we walked into the ultrasound unit for our next scan. On ultrasound, the fetal bowel appeared white rather than the usual soft grey, referred to in obstetrics as *echogenic fetal bowel.* The loops of intestine were in fact as bright as the nearby bones themselves. The amniotic fluid volume was also abnormally high. A fetal CMV infection was now raging, with the abdomen the primary battleground but combat potentially ongoing anywhere, even the brain. The sonographer scanned carefully back and forth through the cranium; the neurologic structures all appeared normal. We may sometimes see direct findings of injury to the fetal brain, none of which were present that day. Thus, it was possible the brain remained uninfected, though it was also possible for CMV to be there already, just not yet visualized, or the brain might be spared only momentarily, with the virus ascending at any moment upward from the abdomen.

Back at home, our two older kids played through the house, unaware of a darkness engulfing their parents as they talked in the kitchen. Once you see findings of fetal infection on ultrasound, most but not all neonates are ultimately diagnosed with some limitation to their health; our overall chances were now worse than a coin flip. We discussed possible outcomes, ranging from hearing loss alone to severe disability to the virus still sparing the brain completely, though our optimism was failing fast as every dice roll after the next had turned against us. As two doctors we would at least be as prepared as one could be for a child with complicated needs. But more than anything I could not shake the overwhelming sense of unfairness. We had already experienced our terrifying first pregnancy, in which emergency surgery was needed at seventeen weeks for a torsed ovarian mass, so following our relatively uncomplicated second delivery, we presumed that future gestations would be uneventful. At that time, we also believed my wife had contracted CMV from her patient, which felt cruel: a punishment for her dedication to children with cancer. For all the good they do, all the sadness and funerals and long nights they face, pediatric oncologists in a beneficent universe would in return live carefree, gilded lives. Of course, in any beneficent universe, there would also be no need for pediatric oncologists.

But what now was the appropriate management? If we remained adherent to our ideology, if we unequivocally believed new interventions to be experimental prior to randomized trials, then we would still recommend against hyperimmune globulin—even if the bowel is brightly echogenic, even if the fluid is increased, even if this is now our own family, with us staring into our own future.

To this day, I ascribe to and practice in accordance with evidence-based medicine, though I must also always acknowledge the adoption of a belief system as the adoption of a belief system, even when based upon science or statistics rather than theology or faith. All have commonalities despite disparate roots, including an oversimplification of future decisions after the original choice to adopt the system itself. For example, say that as a physician I adopt a certain epistemic threshold that must be met prior to me recommending any new treatment—a threshold such as the existence of randomized trials. Then if I wished, all my future patient care decisions could also be collapsed into the same threshold. The decision process may still be time and labor-intensive, requiring that I delve deeply and skeptically into the medical literature, search through research, distinguish between study methodologies, and then at the end throw all I have found against my adopted epistemic belief. At the annual MFM conference, like-minded colleagues and I attend lectures and poster sessions—reviewing the prior year's new research, debating which treatments now lie on which side of the thresholds, and later returning home on airplanes armed with updated clinical recommendations. Each time you then make a decision for a patient, you will tell yourself you are somehow not really responsible; the responsibility lies instead with the existing body of medical knowledge, the epistemic lines, the existence or absence of randomized trials, but not *you*.

But of course, this is never really true; the premise was instantly phantasmal when we sat in a dark room looking at our own ultrasound. Although we may prefer to pass over to our adopted beliefs the reigns of our responsibility, then to be carted passively down roads more treacherous when transversed on foot, we never truly surrender the reins. Lying in the drawn cart is always a fantastical daydream; the reigns are still held when we are forced to look into our hands and are never felt so tightly as when the decisions now weigh against us or those we love. The decisions we make are never from within our systems, but from within our lives and our relationships.

If, at that moment, we still chose to forgo the hyperimmune globulin, was that truly the best choice, or was I in actuality stubborn, obstinate, a zealotry ideologue, or, perhaps worse, a martyr by proxy? It was not lost on me that if we held strong and everything then ended well, I could forever hold my head high among fellow adherents to evidence-based medicine, having not wavered an inch in a moment of personal darkness. When patients asked the unavoidable though usually unanswerable question, "What would you do if this were your wife?" I could then respond proudly and free of hypotheticals. Likewise, if I advocated instead for hyperimmune globulin, I would be forever a hypocrite, the politician who rallies loudly against abortion then supports a loved one facing suddenly perilous circumstances.

Ultimately, there is always just the decision you make. We did not request hyperimmune globulin.

When our daughter was born, her physical examination was perfectly normal, including her hearing screen. An amniocentesis after the ultrasound with the echogenic bowel had not detected the virus, though there is a known false negative rate in this context. However, we soon discovered she still harbored and was fighting CMV; the virus was present when tested in the urine from her diaper and seen under the microscope in the placenta. There remained no evidence of neurologic infection, though; the imaging of her brain was reassuring. Delayed cognitive impacts, including hearing loss, remained possible, with a full two years of monitoring in front of us, so we had to remain settled in, waiting, hopeful.

Two years later my daughter remained completely healthy. Over a decade later, she excels in school, loves to read, joined the archery club, and launches arrows into bull's-eyes. She has read many of the chapters of this book, including this one, giving me her thoughts and feedback. The randomized trial of hyperimmune globulin, meanwhile, continued for years after her birth, as endeavors of this magnitude are as labor-intensive as they are critical. Upon later moving to Cleveland, our hospital was a participating study site, and I became the satellite site investigator who, along with hundreds of others, helped enroll participants. Finally, in 2021, the completed study was published, also in the *New England Journal of Medicine*.[6] For pregnant patients with CMV, hyperimmune globulin held no benefit at all. The rate of the primary outcome of congenital infection or perinatal death occurred in 22.7 percent of participants receiving hyperimmune globulin versus 19.4 percent of those unknowingly receiving a placebo, results that are statistically equivalent, indicating the antibodies had, in fact, no value greater than a sterile bag of salt water.

The results are, of course, fundamentally more depressing than validating as regardless of ideology, everyone would have preferred that hyperimmune globulin actually helped patients with CMV. Research continues, with the future cautiously optimistic. In 2020, a randomized trial in the *Lancet* demonstrated reduced placental passage among patients given the antiviral valacyclovir.[7] Of course, it is always preferable to avoid infections in the first place, and promising trials of CMV vaccination also are underway.

As this is an area of ongoing evolution, any pregnant patient with a CMV exposure or infection should talk to their obstetric provider about current management. At the time of writing, however, there sadly still exist no standard treatments for congenital CMV. For many patients with severe infections, especially those with ultrasound evidence of neurologic injury, abortion may be considered. However, most bans make no exceptions for TORCH. So how can pregnant patients in restrictive states avoid CMV?

Months after our daughter was born, we discovered that my wife had contracted the virus not actually from her patient, which is uncommon for healthcare workers, but likely from our older children in daycare. The major risk factor for CMV, in fact, is being pregnant while simultaneously having another child in a daycare center that has an outbreak. Thus, prevention strategies center upon avoiding household contact with bodily secretions. Of course, avoiding the secretions of your toddler is easier advised than achieved. The National CMV Foundation has five commonsense precautions for childcare while simultaneously pregnant, including washing your hands after changing diapers and avoiding saliva by kissing your baby on the forehead rather than the lips.[8] One of the five recommendations, *do not place a pacifier in your mouth*, may give a reader pause; it raises the question of why a sane adult would ever put their baby's pacifier in their own mouth in the first place. However, parenthood can be a disorienting experience in which you essentially cannot rule out any behavior. And particularly for those living in states with bans, we are often just left doing the things we are able to do.

9 BLEEDING: MISCARRIAGE, HEMORRHAGE, AND PLACENTAL ABRUPTION

In November 2024, ProPublica reported the death of Porsha Ngumezi,[1] one of the small though quickly growing number of patients known to have died under abortion bans. With her husband, she had three- and five-year-old sons at home when she was again pregnant, this time hoping for a girl. However, at ten weeks she began to bleed, progressively passing larger clots until she presented to the emergency department at Houston Methodist Sugar Land Hospital on June 11, 2023. There she continued bleeding, now with clots the size of grapefruit. Her medical records were later reviewed for ProPublica by over a dozen physicians who unanimously agreed that she urgently needed a dilation and curettage procedure, known as a D&C, to evacuate the uterine contents and stop the bleeding. But a D&C was not performed. It was not performed as she continued to hemorrhage, as she passed out, as she received blood transfusions and was moved into the ICU, as she died. Why did she not receive the procedure that would have saved her life? Formally, we do not know as the hospital and managing obstetrician have not spoken in detail publicly. However, it is certainly plausible that the D&C could have been perceived as an abortion under Texas law. In theory, her case should have been entirely unrelated to abortion, as this was a desired pregnancy in someone who had not sought abortion care, but often the lines separating miscarriage and abortion are quite indistinct, especially if criminal jeopardy is in the balance.

But even if the procedure would have formally constituted an abortion, why would it still not have been performed before she died? Would abortion in this case have not been justified under an affirmative defense? Likewise, could this happen even in a state without abortion bans? One of the fundamental problems with bleeding is that it is often ambiguous in magnitude; it lacks uniform definitions and criteria. One would intuitively think bleeding in medicine would always be exactly defined—and in the operating room, performing surgery, we can formally quantify blood loss by measuring suction canisters and weighing sponges. But that is a specific, controlled setting. What about bleeding that occurs at home or elsewhere in the real world or is ongoing while a patient sits in the emergency department? This is not only an obstetrics quandary but one also of trauma, gastroenterology, and any area of medicine in which patients bleed. For example, say that a patient reports a few drops of blood identified when wiping. Does that qualify as "bleeding"? If not, then how much blood is needed? And if a patient bleeds at home, how do you numerically quantify that blood loss? Often we are left listening closely to the description: How much was in the toilet, on the floor, or soaked into garments? Like a crime scene, I examine cell phone photographs or articles of clothing from a plastic bag.

One way to measure blood loss, of course, would be to look for signs of anemia: pallor, an accelerating heart rate, falling blood pressure, dizziness. However, our goal is for these changes to never occur, for physicians to intervene and stop the bleeding, by performing an abortion if necessary, well before this point. The patient whose heart has started to race, whose blood pressure has started to fall, whose consciousness has started to fade, is also the patient who is dying, the patient for which everything may already be too late—a patient like those who have died after Dobbs.

Bleeding's definitional quandaries have long hindered researchers. Years ago, a colleague and I published a meta-analysis of bleeding in pregnancy.[2] In a meta-analysis, a researcher comprehensively searches the medical literature for all known publications on a given topic, then statistically amalgamates the studies into a bird's-eye view of our total knowledge. The papers we searched for were cohorts of typical, healthy, pregnant patients to see how often they experienced bleeding and, if bleeding did occur, how great of a risk it then posed. What we found was that studies varied widely in their conflicting definitions of *bleeding* and, by corollary, how many patients were then said to bleed. For example, one study may define *bleeding* very strictly as a blood loss sufficient for a hospital admission. In that study, few patients had this degree of bleeding, but those who did faced sizable risks. Another study, alternatively, may consider even the smallest loss to be bleeding. In that publication, sizable swaths of their patients had bleeding, though the bleeding, being often more trivial, endeavored few if any risks at all. Thus in the final meta-analysis, when we sought to answer questions such as "How many pregnant patients have bleeding?" or "How risky is bleeding?" by reviewing the amassed medical literature, we saw only a heterogeneous mess, with clear conclusions impeded by the wide range of study results.

Before Dobbs, these definitional concerns haunted academics researching obstetric bleeding. Now the same questions haunt general clinicians with bleeding patients under abortion bans. How do we define bleeding, and how do we then determine the risk relative to restrictive laws? How do we stop Porsha Ngumezi from dying? Formal, legal answers will vary by state. Ohio's abortion ban included bleeding as one of the five exceptions. It did not fall under an affirmative defense but was a listed exception—but it was also just that one word, *bleeding*. However, every state should have some avenue to intervene prior to death.

Why, in the first place, do patients bleed? Most often, bleeding originates from the placenta itself, referred to after mid-pregnancy as *placental abruption*. Abruption has many risk factors, including hypertension and tobacco use. It can also occur after trauma—in particular, motor vehicle accidents whose impact directly shears the placenta from the uterine wall. Sometimes, like almost everything in obstetrics, it can occur randomly in healthy patients. When it occurs randomly, we wonder why, though perhaps a better question would be why it does not occur all the time given the placenta's enormous blood flow.

Early in development, the placenta invades the uterus's endometrial lining to establish a blood supply, though it has to somehow invade exactly deep enough for a vascular connection but not so deeply that it cannot then, at the conclusion of pregnancy, quickly and entirely detach to exit the body. Sometimes this balance is not struck, with the placenta invading excessively and then remaining entrapped in the uterus after delivery, a condition called an *accreta*. Accretas are a significant cause of obstetric hemorrhage, with their early identification also a scenario in which abortion is considered. Alternatively, rather than invading too deeply, a placental portion may fail to remain coterminous and partially detach. In later pregnancy, an enormous volume of blood flows constantly through the uterus—over a half liter per minute, constituting 10 percent of the body's total cardiac output.[3] The placenta must be attached firmly enough that no blood ever leaks out, which would be an abruption, but not so firmly that it does not detach completely after delivery, which would be an accreta. Although we often do not know the cause of a given patient's abruption, it is also amazing that they do not occur more often than they do.

Abruptions occur at a range of gestational ages and severities. If a patient has an abruption at term, then we deliver the fetus. If the patient is preterm, we balance the abruption's severity against the gestational age if delivered. If it is prior to viability, then we weigh these same risks against abortion. In no case, however, does a doctor have much ability to mitigate the bleeding itself. Because abruptions can occur randomly in any pregnancy in any state at any time, a bleeding, previable patient may walk into any emergency room in any state at any moment. Thus, abruption is central to the litigation that has erupted after Dobbs regarding emergency management.

The Emergency Medical Treatment and Labor Act (EMTALA) was passed by congress in 1986 and details the management of emergency care in hospitals that accept Medicare. A person believing themselves to have an emergency is required to receive, at minimum, an evaluation called a medical screening examination (MSE) to determine if a medical emergency exists. If the MSE determines that there is no actual medical emergency, then the patient no longer falls under EMTALA regulations. If an emergency does exist, then the hospital is required to provide care in accordance with their ability to do so. If the patient requires treatments that are not available at that hospital, then they can be transferred to an alternate facility; otherwise, if treatment is available, then it must be provided where they are until the patient is stabilized.

For example, say that a truck strikes a woman driving along a rural road, fracturing her leg. Her femur requires an orthopedic procedure, optimally performed expediently as the damage is ongoing. The ambulance takes her to the nearest emergency department, but that facility has no orthopedic surgeon on staff. America's smaller hospitals rarely have all available services; not every hospital can offer everything, but these limitations are outweighed by their existence in the rural community in the first place. For example, smaller hospitals usually do not have advanced neonatal care, requiring that preterm patients arriving with labor, PPROM, or other complications be transferred to larger facilities. Increasingly, many rural hospitals have no labor and delivery department at all as units are closing throughout the United States, leaving vacuums in their wakes. Likewise, in this example of the broken leg, the woman would need to be transferred to the nearest orthopedist.

But what if the rural hospital did have a surgeon on staff, but they just didn't want to operate on the driver's leg? Before EMTALA, this occurred frequently—sometimes for explicitly racist reasons, such as when "white" hospitals would turn away Black patients. But often surgeons would decline for financial reasons, such as the patient being uninsured or having public insurance that reimbursed at a lower rate. However, for this woman, the risks to her leg are increasing with time, and the best medical course is to have surgery now at the current hospital without being transported away. This is where EMTALA factors in: The hospital cannot transfer without consent for any procedure that is both emergent and locally available. Under EMTALA, the orthopedist drives to the hospital and changes into scrubs.

The next day, another truck strikes a car along the same road, and the driver again is taken to the same hospital. This time the driver is pregnant at twenty weeks gestation, and rather than a broken leg, she has a placental abruption. Depending upon the degree of hemorrhage, an urgent abortion may be needed to save her life. However, if the hospital has no obstetricians or gynecologists, then transfer to a larger hospital may be needed. The transfer would carry risks, including just the time spent moving between facilities, but sometimes in medicine there are no perfect options.

What if the hospital had a gynecologist who could perform the procedure, but they didn't want to operate and instead wanted the patient to be transferred away? Perhaps this physician holds personal beliefs. Or maybe they support reproductive freedoms but are reasonably terrified, fearing criminal liability under a ban that relegates saving a life to only an affirmative defense. Does EMTALA still apply? This is the fundamental question right now before our courts and legislative leaders. Like the woman the day before, this patient needs a procedure and the hospital can provide the procedure, so the appropriate course is treatment at the current location without transfer. Why should anything be different if the treatment happens to be abortion? And if EMTALA does not apply, then how is this not a direct endangerment on the basis of pregnancy and sex?

Questions surrounding abortion bans and EMTALA began almost immediately after Dobbs. If a patient presented to an emergency department needing abortion care, a doctor right now could find themselves trapped between their state ban and federal EMTALA legislation. At the time of writing, these questions are being litigated before the United States Supreme Court. Pending resolution, many states currently do not recognize EMTALA with regard to their own bans.

Therefore, many physicians potentially could legally transfer an endangered patient they could otherwise treat. However, what is or is not legal is never equivalent to what we should or should not do. Ethically, are you required to care for the patient regardless of the law? Do physicians have no choice in to whom we provide care, the patients we do or do not see? Or are we the medical equivalent of a waiter in a restaurant, never able to control who does or does not walk through the doors?

One evening, a patient I never personally cared for arrived at our emergency department after being struck by a car. Her severe injuries spanned multiple organs and bones. The impact also sheered the placenta in a catastrophic abruption, with the fetal heart rate decelerating downward as the uterus swelled with blood. As she was preterm but not previable, the obstetrics team performed an emergent cesarean right in the trauma bay, but they were too late; the outcome was likely inevitable before the patient even entered the unit's doors, with the neonate not surviving.

That night, while the obstetrics and trauma surgeons desperately operated, the police arrested the car's driver, who was subsequently charged with attempted murder, a less typical accusation in such scenarios as murder implies intent, whereas automotive traumas are usually accidental. In this case, however, the authorities did not believe anything to be accidental as the driver was a romantic rival simultaneously pregnant by the same partner.

After the cesarean, the trauma patient faced a long recovery with orthopedic and plastic procedures, followed likely by extensive physical therapy; she would likely struggle initially to rise out of her hospital bed. The obstetrics team continued to round through much of her stay, well past the surgical healing from the abruption itself, monitoring her both physically and through her grief. Authorities, meanwhile, initially held the driver after her arrest, then charged her and released her on bail. Prosecutors didn't want to risk her trial being disrupted by the pregnancy—as it might be, for example, if she began laboring during a deposition. They decided instead for her to remain free until after delivery, scheduling the criminal proceedings for months after her due date. Thus, on a subsequent weekday, with the abruption patient still recovering and grieving upstairs, the driver walked into the same hospital's offices for a routine prenatal visit.

The ethical conundrum was debated throughout the city's obstetric community. Many of the residents on call that night for the trauma requested not to provide care to the driver after all they had witnessed. While one patient struggled through rehabilitation, learning to walk on fractured bones, the other strolled into our clinic, where doctors measured her expanding belly with a paper ruler. Further complicating matters, the father often accompanied the driver to her visits. The driver would sit in the ultrasound suite, her partner dutifully seated at her side, happily watching a healthy fetus on the screen in black and white.

Despite discomfort, or perhaps even moral anguish, the predominant view was that the driver still deserved care. First, there was the technical matter of one being innocent until proven guilty—here likely just a formality as the facts were as clear as they were disquieting, with the driver striking the other woman directly where she stood and causing the abruption. But regardless, we were still committed to care, both legally and professionally. Even if we did not want to, we would have been bound by EMTALA had the driver walked into our unit in labor. Thus, her physicians and nurses buried deep and then provided care, doing so politely if not perhaps bitterly.

A waiter in a restaurant stands before a tray intended for a bespectacled gentleman and his life partner. Does he pick up the tray and carry it to the table? To do so is required by a waiter's condition of employment, though it would be dangerously disingenuous to say he does not then have a choice; we always have choices. But the delivery of the tray represents the irreducible essence of being a waiter. He remains free to walk away instead; waiters in the real world often quit, often for justifiable reasons. Maybe his wages are too low or his objections ethical, the entree roast veal from a restricted calf or the patrons rumored to have seduced students at the Lycée Molière. The choice to carry or not carry the tray, however, is not independent from that of being or not being a waiter. Despite the enormity of our freedom, one nevertheless cannot choose to both refuse the tray and remain a waiter.

When the driver began to labor, arriving at the hospital for delivery, what choices faced those healthcare workers that day? The final, irreducible essence of medicine is care. Physicians can also choose to walk away instead. They can work for insurance companies or become administrators. They can enter other fields or even become legislators themselves. But the decision to remain a doctor is the decision to provide care—even when you face a criminal risk, even when you disagree on matters of reproduction, even when your patient commits a crime or has struck down another woman with her car. In medicine, we care for both the injured innocent and the injurious incarcerated. So as the driver labored in her room, her fetus on the heart rate monitor, the contractions ebbing and receding, the team provided care—perhaps with a congratulations that rang hallow, perhaps with smiles forcibly stretched over gritted teeth. Usually in medicine, care lies in our center, draped under performative layers of jargon, scrubs, and white coats. That evening, care was instead the performance, itself now wrapped over a smoldering, angry core.

Her delivery was uncomplicated, and she left the hospital a few days later, her healthy child wrapped warmly in her arms. After that, months went by, and I forgot about the case given my absence of direct involvement, the story's unpleasant nature, and the unending flow of new and complicated patients. One day, as I loitered in the break room awaiting the start of surgery, I happened to glance an article in the local newspaper, lying obliquely on the central table. The driver at trial had been found innocent on the basis of self-defense. Now wildly curious, I grabbed the paper and read the story of what actually happened that night.

The two women had been in obvious conflict, centered around the common father, which came to a head that evening when one organized a group of friends to confront the other. The intended target, however, was the future driver sitting in her home unaware; the organizer was the future abruption patient who, with compatriots, breeched the woman's house with presumed malicious intent. The homeowner, terrified, fled through the back into the driveway, where her car sat parked, with the other woman and her friends in close pursuit. She entered and locked the car's doors, though not before being surrounded, engulfed by shouting, hands rocking the frame, and the other woman standing, with her protruding abdomen, in front, blocking her exit. She had to make a decision, like we all so often do, with just the information she had and time running out. Was her life that night really in danger? Was their intent really to harm or to just frighten and harass? Was the other woman bluffing by standing in front of her car, or would she move? Ultimately, she made the decision to press the gas pedal, driving a tragic distance before hearing the screams of someone trapped under the car being dragged through the street.

This full story had been unknown through her pregnancy while she was on bail awaiting trial. But certainly, she must have told the police her version upon arrest. Did they not believe her that night? Was her story not corroborated? I don't know, though these questions also don't really matter as self-defense, like many physicians right now providing abortion to save a patient's life, is affirmative, such that the driver was still charged to later, under her own burden, prove self-defense. She was ultimately acquitted, though with criminal charges hanging over her head for months otherwise spent trying to enjoy her pregnancy, the delivery, and then her child.

After my surprise reading the story, my next reaction was relief that the team caring for her had still done so. Although she was not physically the victim herself, her experience nevertheless must have been traumatic. Did she ponder her responsibility, her choice, the alternative universe where she did not step on the gas? When she held her healthy child, could she suppress the vision of the other woman's loss?

But what of the other woman, the trauma patient? What if that night, as she was rushed in on a stretcher, bleeding, abrupting, in critical condition, every doctor and nurse somehow already knew the entire story—that she was in fact the alleged perpetrator? The concept of justice is powerful, though ultimately abstract. The patient in front of you is always real. Would anything actually have changed for the healthcare workers that night? Would they have not still desperately performed a cesarean? Stop her bleeding, repair her bones, save her life? Would they have not listened to her weep?

Pregnant patients right now in states with abortion bans should know which hospitals they can go to in the event of an emergency and what care that hospital is legally required to provide. Often ambulances will take patients to the physically closest hospital regardless of whether or not that facility actually can serve their need. Thus, a pregnant patient in an ambulance should always ask if they are being taken to a hospital that has obstetric services—specifically, a labor and delivery unit—and if not, why not. Because emergencies can occur unexpectedly, you should know the current status of EMTALA in your state. If someone is facing a threat to their health that may require abortion, they should ask if a physician is on staff who can perform abortion; if not, then they may require transfer.

10 STRUCTURE: CONGENITAL ANOMALIES

Structural congenital anomalies, a.k.a. *birth defects*, occur in 3 to 5 percent of all pregnancies.[1] With rare exceptions, they either form or do not form in the first trimester, during a range of weeks called the *teratogenic window*. Once formed in this window, defects may later be repairable surgically, but they will be otherwise fixed embryologically. Unfortunately, many patients are not yet aware of being pregnant in the early teratogenic window, resulting in unintentional exposures, such as alcohol use. Some medications also increase the risk of birth defects, with thalidomide and diethylstilbestrol the most historic examples. Excessive levels of blood sugar in diabetic patients also can be causative. However, if you take all the medications and drugs and diseases and add them together, you will only account for a minority of birth defects, with the others occurring despite perfect health. Thus anyone can, through random chance, have a structural anomaly; they occur across all backgrounds, economic strata, ages, and geographic locations. You can have no family history, abstain from alcohol, take no medications, be a good person who works to make the world a better place, and there is still a risk.

Truly random risks can be uniquely unsettling, especially when under abortion bans with no exceptions, if not outright prohibitions, for fetal conditions. If a person is considering pregnancy in a restrictive state, then a congenital anomaly is a fixed risk within the decision to conceive. Likewise, some of the earliest, most heartbreaking stories emerging after Dobbs centered on patients forced to continue despite severe birth defects.

In Florida in 2023, Deborah Dorbert was forced to carry to term[2] a fetus with *Potter syndrome*, a condition in which kidneys do not form. In addition to just the absence of the kidneys themselves, there is also no amniotic fluid as this is made by the fetal renal system. The absence of fluid in turn leads to severe pulmonary hypoplasia, such that fetuses are then born with neither functioning kidneys nor lungs. Florida at the time had a fifteen-week ban; it is now even more unforgiving at six weeks. For Dorbert, the birth defects were not identified until after fifteen weeks, which is quite usual; given the smaller fetal size before then, most are not seen prior to that point. Also typical was the fact that she was healthy with an earlier uncomplicated pregnancy, a four-year-old son playing through their house. She and her husband had chosen to conceive again; they wanted more children and had no reason to foresee what they subsequently endured. After receiving the diagnosis, Dorbert's physicians stated she could attempt to escape Florida for care elsewhere, but she did not have the financial ability to do so. She was instead forced to embark on an agonizing thirteen-week journey, all along knowing exactly what lay at the end. As the weeks went by, she became increasingly depressed,[3] lying on the couch, feeling the fetal movement; she later entered marriage counseling with her husband. In Potter syndrome, there is no amniotic fluid, so the mother continuously feels every movement; the uterine wall is draped about every fetal limb without buffer. Their four-year-old son was aware of the pregnancy and became excited about his new sibling, but they could not forever hide what was going to happen from him. They named their child Milo, and when Milo was born, they held him while he died, moving his chest but unable to breathe. Although she had always planned a larger family, Dorbert said to reporters she was now unsure of ever becoming pregnant again.

Stories such as these prevent birth defects from descending into cold science and facts. Congenital anomalies in particular are researched through a wide array of disciplines. Embryologists study organ formation, pharmacologists the teratogenic risks, environmentalists the impact of pollution, and epidemiologists the clustering of cases. Birth defects are debated by ethicists and legal scholars. Pollsters track public attitudes toward abortion for structural anomalies. But all these layers of inquiry should never obstruct what lies at the center: the experience of the patient for whom a birth defect is diagnosed. How much, after all, can something be understood by researching it?

Do I, for example, understand labor as a male physician? When my wife was in labor with our second child, one of my responsibilities was music. Pandora was relatively novel at that time, so I sat in a chair rummaging through songs and artists. Having been a college DJ, this felt like the ultimate challenge of musical curation, so I mixed classics like Cat Stevens and Joan Baez with Mazzy Star, Lambchop, Jimmie Dale Gilmore, and the wonderful Magnetic Fields. A success: We would play the channel for weeks after around the house with our infant son. Thus, when my wife entered labor with our third child, I sprung again into my role; that pregnancy in particular was stressful on account of the CMV infection and agonizing decisions regarding intravenous immunoglobulins.

Sitting in the labor room, her contractions would come and go in waves, swelling over a few seconds, during which she would close her eyes and breathe deeply, then retreat as the uterine muscles relaxed, after which the waters would still for a few minutes until the next wave arrived. That was when inspiration struck for the perfect genre choice for labor: surf music, like the ocean waves themselves. Surf music had enjoyed a brief though thrilling revival in the 1990s. In 1994, the *Pulp Fiction* soundtrack featured the great Dick Dale performing "Misirlou," originally a Mediterranean folk song. It felt perfect that day. Not just the metaphor of ocean waves but the genre's inherent energy matching the gravity of the event. I concentrated during the interlude between contractions on finding the perfect surf song. Then, as the next contraction began to swell, with my wife again closing her eyes and breathing deeply, so began a rolling, opening baseline, building in excitement through the peak and continuing as the contraction abated. My wife was then able to open her eyes again and speak to me.

It turns out that surf music during labor is actually a terrible choice. If you are reading this as a future labor support person, play euphonious and mellifluous music; definitely do not play rambling, jangling surf music.

My unfortunate genre selection that day did not stem from any lack of factual knowledge regarding labor, for which I had tremendous medical expertise. At that time, I had studied labor in textbooks for hours, delivered uncounted babies, and, in the laboratory, analyzed uterine muscle cells in culture dishes bathed in nutrient-rich media. I had lectured on labor to residents and fellows, published scientific papers in peer-reviewed journals. But did I understand labor as an actual, lived experience?

As a medical student, I had likewise been drawn to studying birth defects. This was primarily, of course, for reasons of patient care. However, if my younger self had been forced to be completely truthful, he would also uncomfortably admit to being mesmerized by the ultrasound images of anomalies. The conjoint twins, the hands of ectrodactyly cleaved through the middle, the normally internal organs floating instead in the fluid outside the body. Dense medical textbooks would overflow with pictures of strange anomalies. In middle school, I was infatuated for a time with the surrealist painter Salvador Dalí, once receiving a large coffee table book of his paintings for Christmas. Years later in medical school, while reading through a textbook about birth defects, I could imagine this was again Dalí as I perused page after page of images and ultrasounds.

But back in middle school, I was just an adolescent fascinated by melting clocks and dreamlike, abstracted figures while blind to Dalí's underlying emotions and motivations. One of my favorite Dalí paintings was *Soft Construction with Boiled Beans (Premonition of Civil War)*, which featured a tangled and twisted body painfully grasping its multiple misplaced limbs. Ogling the painting, I was entirely unaware of its underlying story, despite *civil war* being right there in the title. Dalí painted it in 1936, a mere six months before war rendered apart his beloved Spain. In the subsequent year, he would flee with his wife to Paris, leaving behind their home to be destroyed, their family and friends to be imprisoned and tortured, and a dear colleague executed by firing squad. In 1936, when Dalí placed his brush against canvas to render this frightful figure, he was under the disquiet of growing unrest. As he drew his inspiration from dreams, this painting is the literal projection of a nightmare. But when I flipped through my book as a kid, I didn't even know of the Spanish Civil War. When I look at this art now, I can see beyond the uncanny figure to the real fear and pain Dalí experienced.

As a medical student flipping through a textbook of fetal anomalies, you don't at first see the underlying stories or consider that each image in the book represents a real pregnancy occurring in a real person who then faced painful choices. Years after school, as a new physician, a sonographer will come into the reading room after identifying an anomaly. You would sit in front of the computer flipping through the images, after which you would now need to walk down the hall to talk to the patient, who at that moment was likely unsuspecting. Suddenly you think less of embryology or genetics or the chemistry of teratogenesis and more of what is about to happen when you walk into that room, introduce yourself, clear your throat. Other times in high-risk obstetrics, we see patients who are themselves adult survivors of fetal birth defects—not only transcending the abstract images we see on machines but here as actual adults talking to you. Perhaps they have a repaired neural tube defect or are living a happy, well-rounded life with an ectrodactylous hand.

When I diagnose fetal anencephaly, however, I know that it will never result in an adult one day talking to me in my office. *Anencephaly* is a severe birth defect in which there is no cranium or cerebral matter above the brainstem; its name is a combination of the Greek roots *an-*, meaning "without," and *cephaly*, referencing the head and brain. There is a spinal column and face, usually with unaltered eyes and nose, but the cranium itself is absent such that nothing else exists from slightly above the eyebrows. It is a variant of neural tube defects, similar to spina bifida, but afflicting the brain resting atop the spine rather than the lower back at the other end. Anencephaly is rare, though not so uncommon that high-risk obstetricians do not still see it many times. I find myself diagnosing it about once or twice a year.

Anencephaly appears frequently in abortion discourse as it is unequivocally lethal. In conversations surrounding anomalies, abortion opponents will often raise the possibility of the doctors being wrong, the prognosis not as bad as described, the chance of survival low but not absolutely zero. PPROM at previable gestational ages, for example, has rare though existent healthy deliveries. For anencephaly, however, there is no such debate. Be it fetal, pediatric, or adult, there probably exists little in medicine as certain as anencephaly. With anencephaly, you do not ponder odds or wonder if you will toss a die or a coin into the air, as when you open your fingers there is only ever your hand. Thus, it is a powerful reference point in conversations about abortion for fetal conditions, though such use also risks anencephaly becoming an argumentative strategy behind which one may not then see actual patients—the policy equivalent of only looking at the pictures in a book.

When I had to tell my first patient that their fetus had anencephaly, in theory I should have been perfectly prepared. I had previously reviewed it in textbooks, studied its embryologic mechanisms, and was well-practiced in delivering terrible diagnoses: You sit in a chair. You make eye contact. You first deliver the essential facts clearly, without a circuitous windup. Then you pause, give them the chance to absorb and react; you sit quietly for a moment as they begin to sob and then ask why this is happening to them. However, anencephaly always feels different. I employ all the standard methods, but I do not know if it helps; maybe it does and the reactions would otherwise be even worse, or maybe the optimal method to convey this exact diagnosis just does not exist. With any of an array of approaches, with all the empathy you can provide, still ultimately you have to tell them that the fetus has no skull, no brain. How do you tell this patient? A patient who is healthy, without risk factors, their pregnancy uneventful to date, excitedly arriving at the unit that day with their loved ones.

When my kids were young and we would go to the zoo on warm weekend days, there would be legions of families there also with small children. As a busy obstetrician, I would look out among the crowd and wonder, statistically, with how many of these families I may have previously crossed paths. How many kids laughing as they feed giraffes I might have seen before on their ultrasounds or helped their parents through their pregnancies. Then I would remember how often my wife or I deliver horrible news, how many times I've diagnosed miscarriage, stillbirth, or anomalies, let alone what she has had to tell families. I wonder how many parents that day at the zoo would, through no specific fault of our own, have hoped to never in their lives see one or the other of us again. Perhaps a former patient or parent labored through a process of grief for years, struggling to find their peace. Then on an amiable summer day, among the elephants and ice cream cones, they look across to my wife or I and are suddenly back again in that moment to which they had never wanted to return.

In the ongoing case of *Zurawski v. State of Texas*, many of the plaintiffs had pregnancies that were complicated by life-limiting anomalies, including several cases of anencephaly itself. In July 2023, three of the plaintiffs testified before the Travis County Civil District Court. One was the suit's namesake, Amanda Zurawski, who had experienced PPROM at eighteen weeks and was later admitted in sepsis to the ICU. The two other plaintiffs, Ashley Brandt and Samantha Casiano, both had pregnancies complicated by anencephaly. At the trial, Samantha Casiano described being forced to carry to term, then watching her child die in the delivery room. In the courtroom recounting her story, she became so upset that she vomited right then and there, with her husband Louis rushing to help. A recess was called, after which she courageously continued once she recovered and the staff had cleaned her emesis from the witness stand.

After Dobbs, these are among the stories that most need to be told, though they are also among the most painful to recount. Over and over, patients have come forward. How brave are those who under the harshest of legal and public lights still made the decision to tell stories so deeply personal? It is one thing for doctors to talk in generalizations or use patient scenarios that are composites or hypotheticals, and another for someone to tell their own story while sworn under oath. A stenographer quietly clicks your every word as you describe your child struggling for air, then the fluids in your stomach churn and escape outward. Or from out of your once peaceful life, a reporter now sits in front of you as a technician runs a microphone wire through your clothing against your skin, while you prepare to answer questions nobody would ever want to answer. But these are the stories that obliterate otherwise sterile pontifications of regulations and exceptions and affirmative defenses.

How can patients living in restrictive states mitigate their risks? An increased focus after Dobbs is the earlier ultrasound identification of birth defects, including at the end of the first trimester, allowing for earlier diagnosis and thus care. Abortion for anomalies may still be illegal even early in gestation, though diagnoses in the first trimester allow for the potential time and logistical coordination to travel out of state. Classically, birth defects are identified around eighteen to twenty weeks when the anatomic ultrasound is performed. When I was a medical student, all that could really be seen at twelve to fourteen weeks was the fetal size and cardiac activity, with only the most egregious of anomalies able to be visualized. As technology has advanced, however, we are now able to see more structural features at increasingly early gestational ages. In a recent systematic review, dedicated ultrasounds could identify a bit over one-third of all birth defects prior to fourteen weeks.[4] The defects able to be identified the earliest are also generally the most severe, and so the percentage of anomalies that are life-limiting that can now be detected in the first trimester is even higher. At this time, the practice of early anatomic evaluations is evolving, with geographic variance in availability. However—and in particular for patients living in states with bans, where time may present a crucial barrier in the event of a birth defect—patients should at least inquire into early anatomic evaluation with their obstetric providers.

Shortly after Dobbs, *The New York Times* reported the story of Madison Underwood, whose abortion for a lethal fetal neurologic anomaly was canceled in Tennessee shortly after the law changed, requiring her to travel to Georgia instead.[5] The anomaly had been identified at the traditional second-trimester ultrasound. However, reading the *Times* article now weeks later, it featured a picture of the patient holding an earlier, first-trimester ultrasound image. It was one of the informal keepsakes often given to patients after sonograms, featuring the fetus with the caption, "Hi Mom!" That ultrasound had been performed before Dobbs, before the ban, when she could have legally pursued an abortion without travel. Looking at the picture in the newspaper, albeit obviously as a physician with specific expertise, I clearly saw the neurologic anomaly, the cranial bones flaring out to the side. The information had been there all along.

11 LIGHTENING: PREECLAMPSIA AND HYPERTENSION IN PREGNANCY

Few indications for abortion are as clear as severe preeclampsia prior to viability. Individual patients always make individual decisions, but given the maternal risks and our inability to optimally treat preeclampsia, abortion in this scenario must at least remain immutable from legal exigencies. In Ohio's ban, preeclampsia was a cited exception, but even in states where such an exemption is not spelled out, even in states where all abortions are relegated to an affirmative defense, abortion for severe preeclampsia prior to viability should remain uncontroversial. Fortunately, preeclampsia that is both severe and prior to fetal viability is rare. Preeclampsia itself, however, is not uncommon across the totality of gestational ages, with its prevalence both increasing and disproportionate over racial and ethnic groups.[1] Its incidence and disparities were particularly highlighted in the 2010s, when several celebrities suffered preeclampsia; socioeconomic status does not convey immunity from this disease. In 2011, worsening preeclampsia forced Mariah Carey to deliver her twins prematurely after her body had swollen with extracellular fluid; she later stated in interviews that she had lost over forty pounds of water after giving birth.[2] In 2018, Beyoncé described her experience with preeclampsia to *Vogue* magazine.[3] More recently and most tragically, the decorated Olympian sprinter Tori Bowie, winner of bronze, silver, and gold metals just a few years before, died from complications of preeclampsia in 2023.[4]

What exactly is preeclampsia? At its most definitional, *preeclampsia* is hypertension that occurs or worsens in the latter half of pregnancy. In medicine, some diseases are clinically defined, meaning that rather than being diagnosed by a single, straightforward laboratory test—for example, bacteria growing in a petri dish or a cell viewed under the microscope—patients are diagnosed according to an agreed-upon constellation of clinical signs and symptoms. Preeclampsia is one such clinically defined disease, such that diagnostic criteria exist as set forth by professional organizations that detail laboratory, gestational age, history, and blood pressure requirements. These criteria evolve over time with changing research and clinical opinions, though for preeclampsia they always entail increasing blood pressures in the latter half of pregnancy.

Beyond blood pressure, preeclampsia can impact a range of organs in the body through capillary leak, with extracellular fluid accumulating in various tissues outside the vascular tree. Patients then classically have edematous ankles and legs, often with swelling of the fingers and face as well. This likely accounts for all the water weight Mariah Carey reported after delivering her twins. Leakage from renal capillaries allows protein to escape into the urine, a condition called *proteinuria* that is strongly associated with the disease. Vascular changes can impact the lungs, the liver, and even the brain itself. The word *eclampsia* describes the seizures that occur when preeclampsia affects the brain, etymologically derived from the Greek noun for lightning and described by Hippocrates himself. Although eclampsia has been known since antiquity, we only discovered the blood pressure elevations and proteinuria that predate the seizures in more modern times—specifically, after the invention of the mercury manometer in the late 1800s allowed physicians to record blood pressure. The changes in blood pressure and urine that would precede the eclamptic seizures was thus called *preeclampsia*. Preeclampsia then over time became the name of the underlying disease itself, making for the unusual semantics of naming a disease with *pre-* followed by one of its severe side effects.

Preeclampsia's human suffering is enormous. The CDC estimates that 6.3 percent of pregnancy-related deaths in America are caused by hypertensive disorders in pregnancy,[5] which furthermore play at least some role in 31.6 percent of inpatient obstetric deaths. Because many patients with preeclampsia require premature delivery, it is also in turn a leading cause of preterm birth. Our treatments against preeclampsia remain limited; intravenous magnesium prevents some seizures, and antihypertensive medications can lower the blood pressure. These have been our same basic tools since I was a medical student, with our field essentially stagnant over the subsequent decades. In fact, many of our improvements in preeclampsia have come from abandoning old treatments now known to be ineffective or even harmful rather than introducing new, efficacious treatments. For example, many generations of physicians treated preeclampsia with strict bedrest on the presumption that lying prone could decrease blood pressure. Beyond preeclampsia, bedrest was prescribed reflexively for a wide range of obstetric complications, such as vaginal bleeding or preterm labor. Like many interventions before and after, it was first deployed on the basis of theory and plausibility, but prior to clinical trials to determine if it was actually effective or even safe. Despite no proof of benefit, bedrest was applied so often that it spurred an entire subgenre of children's literature—books that a mother could hand to older siblings to explain why she was in bed all day, such as *Mommy Has to Stay in Bed* by Annette Rivlin-Gutman, *Bedrest Mommy* by Jennifer Christensen and Mike Boltz, and *Stuck in Bed* by Jennifer Degl and Angela Davids.

Bedrest was often as draconian as it was frequent. Patients would first be hospitalized, then placed prone, then told not to arise. Once I saw a woman for an outpatient visit after she had been discharged from the hospital on strict bedrest. When I inquired into her week she described, to my horror, the details of her routine: uncertain if standing was allowed at all she MacGyvered a system for moving about using an older child's skateboard. When she inevitably needed to go to the bathroom, the kitchen, or elsewhere, she would slide off her bed onto the skateboard, then, with protuberant abdomen and off-kilter balance, transverse hallways by pushing with her legs and pulling with her arms.

We now know that strict bedrest is harmful rather than helpful, in alignment with the general principle that activity is healthy and inactivity is not. Immobility in particular risks blood clots and the wasting of muscle mass. But in retrospect, bedrest was not only medically erroneous but wildly paternalistic. Early in my training, the field of obstetrics was still predominantly male. We would look upon medically endangered pregnant patients, see their vulnerability, then choose to constrain, to constrict. In misguided benevolence, we extracted them from their work or even engagements with the world at large. They would read picture books to older children that explained why they were now medical prisoners. Through the course of pregnancy, a person might transition from autonomy to vulnerability to literal immobilization by physician decree.

But if not through bedrest, then how does one actually stop preeclampsia? Ultimately, the only resolution remains the delivery of the placenta, and thus by corollary the fetus. When preeclampsia occurs at term, then delivery is straightforward; if preterm, the decision can be agonizing as one balances the risks of the disease against the risk of the neonate being premature. And if the patient is so premature as to be previable, then abortion may be necessary. Often, we try to prolong preterm preeclampsia if we can do so safely. Broadly, preeclampsia is divided into the categories of severe and not severe. If not severe, then preeclampsia can be watched until thirty-seven weeks; a case of severe preeclampsia must be delivered in contrast by thirty-four weeks at the latest. Certain manifestations of severe preeclampsia, however, necessitate delivery at any gestational age, including abortion if previable, as conservative management beyond stabilization or steroids for fetal optimization carries unacceptable risks. A list of such contraindications is published by the American College of Obstetricians and Gynecologists and includes kidney dysfunction, stroke, pulmonary edema, and eclamptic seizures themselves. Someone who is or has a loved one with preeclampsia in a restrictive state can consult this list to determine if abortion potentially is being inappropriately withheld.

Optimally, treatments would exist beyond just delivery. Our frustrating inability to treat preeclampsia stems from the fact that, despite years of research, the cause remains fundamentally mysterious. And not just mysterious, but at times perhaps even nonsensical. In MFM, we manage preeclampsia so routinely that we rarely pause to ponder why it exists in the first place. Outside of reports of gorillas seizing in pregnancy, preeclampsia is an exclusively human disease, inexistent in the wider animal kingdom. In fact, one of the frustrating roadblocks to our research is the absence of natural animal models. As preeclampsia likely arises from the placenta, investigators have looked at placental differences compared to other species for an explanatory cause. Among mammals, there exist three fundamental types of placentas, of which ours are *hemochorial*, the least common subtype. However, hemochorial placentas are shared with not only our fellow primates but also rodents. As rodents never seize in pregnancy, our placental subtypes alone cannot then explain preeclampsia. Another theory is that the human brain is disproportionately large relative to other mammals, thus requiring an increased nutrient supply that in turn overburdens our placentas, somehow triggering preeclampsia. However, this is only a theory, with mechanistic lacunae, and one of many theories that exist. Preeclampsia has often been called the *disease of theories*, given the abundance of conjecture relative to our lack of certainty. In the 1800s, physicians coined the expression *toxemia of pregnancy* as they believed preeclampsia to arise from some toxin in the body; their subsequent treatments therefore were bloodletting and purging. In 1983, researchers believed they had found a parasite, *Hydatoxi lualba*, embedded in preeclamptic placentas when viewed through their microscopes, leading to a theory that it was caused by a small worm. However, their "worm" was later discovered to be an erroneous artifact from staining the glass slides.

But more upsetting than just not knowing its cause is the disquieting fact that preeclampsia appears to serve no beneficial purpose. For most diseases, we can construct some story to explain why they exist, even if we wish they did not. With age and repetitive use, our muscles, joints, and tendons wear down, leading to myalgias and arthritis. Bacteria and viruses exist in this world often as our friends, but sometimes are our enemies. Over the trillions of times our cells divide, a mistranslation eventually yields cancer. Carrying a single copy of the genes that cause cystic fibrosis or sickle cell disease protects a person against, respectively, cholera or malaria, explaining their existence from an evolutionary perspective.

Many cases of preterm labor are also explainable: The body has determined that delivery is needed as it believes some problem has arisen. For example, in placental abruption or amniotic infections, the uterus begins to contract, with the goal of protecting the parent and fetus through delivery. Or perhaps MMPs are released, rupturing the fetal membranes. This is why most patients begin to labor after they experience PPROM. Sometimes in cases of preterm labor, we believe the uterine contractions to be mistaken; the patient is premature and we are unable to identify bleeding, inflammation, or another explanation. Thus, we attempt to stop the labor. But then sometimes we discover after delivery that the body was actually right, with an infection or hemorrhage in the placenta later identified microscopically. When a patient arrives prematurely laboring, one of the questions asked before trying to stop it is if, in fact, the body is correct in contracting. We wish preterm labor did not occur, but on a fundamental level it makes sense. We can see the physiologic rationale, even if we disagree.

But why does preeclampsia exist? What is the logic underlying preeclampsia? Unlike abruption or PPROM, patients with preeclampsia will not usually contract in order to deliver. Rather, the disease will just progress onward without resolution, the patient's blood pressure increasing and increasing, until, if left to its own accord, the patient may seize and then die unless physicians or midwives step in to intervene via delivering. The blood pressure elevations themselves have no clear benefit, only harm. What purpose does that serve? What is the positive against which this disease's negatives are balanced? Perhaps our knowledge simply is still limited; maybe one day a rational explanation will be revealed. Often we read authors from the past waxing poetic upon mysteries of their time that are now well-elucidated in the present. Certainly during my career, our understanding of preeclampsia has advanced in concert with the relentless researchers working against it. We better understand the roles of placental trophoblast cells invading into spiral arteries or circulating antiangiogenic factors such as soluble fms-like tyrosine kinase-1. But despite such advancements, the fundamental question of purpose remains unanswered.

In labor and delivery, as a preeclamptic patient's blood pressure climbs terrifyingly, relentlessly upward, as she suffers headaches and visual changes from her brain literally swelling with fluid, she may reasonably ask why this is happening. Be it medical, evolutionary, physiologic, or perhaps even philosophic, I do not have an answer. In a universe that is beneficent, or even just reasonably sensible, preeclampsia should not exist. The blood pressures, the edema, the headaches, the seizures, all appear as suffering without greater purpose. Perhaps one day researchers will find the answers, though at this moment we could make a case for it being, in only the classic, tragic use of the word, *absurd*.

In September 2021, after the Supreme Court failed to block Texas's ban, *Scientific American* published an article titled "The Absurd Pregnancy Math Behind the 'Six-Week' Abortion Ban," which opens with "The law the Supreme Court just failed to block is not just a blow to women; it's biologically nonsensical."[6] The word *absurd* is often used in the context of abortion bans—in particular, those in which a pregnancy is forcibly continued with a life-limiting anomaly. Laws requiring a term delivery when the fetus will only live minutes or hours can feel as deeply illogical as they are cruel. But then are abortion bans, like perhaps preeclampsia, also absurd?

If I traveled back in time to my tenth-grade English class, I would marvel at the juxtaposition of setting, audience, and subject as our cohort of early teens discussed Camus and Beckett from mostly uneventful lives in North Allegheny's quiet Pittsburgh suburb. In class that year, we focused on the early and mid-century literature born from the horrors of the global wars into which authors had found themselves thrown. The concept of absurdity is strongly associated with this period: absurdist fiction, the theatre of the absurd, existentialism, Dadaism. But absurdity dates to at least ancient Greece, if not the dawn of humanity itself. For as long as we have looked out into the world and seen cruelty without apparent cause, suffering without apparent reason, we have contemplated absurdity: the earthquake striking a pious town, a person standing under a falling tree. In medicine, we see absurdity all the time—never of course in a humorous sense, but rather in the ways in which diseases strike randomly, with courses that cannot then be predicted; in watching good people suffer and bad people heal day in and out; in the healthy patient developing severe preeclampsia; in my wife's patient, a child ravaged by cancer.

Abortion bans can be described in many ways: cruel, tyrannical, tortuous, misogynistic. But are they also absurd? They may certainly be irrational, illogical, perhaps even Kafkaesque. In cases of life-limiting fetal anomalies, a forced continuation leads to suffering without purpose. Furthermore, the voting public does not even want this to happen; the ban's very existence is nonsensical in a representative democracy. I will leave to philosophers the question of why patients face suffering itself, but everything surrounding abortion bans, everything surrounding their forced continuation, is clearly laid out in front of us. It is not an earthquake or natural disaster, a pandemic of unknown genesis, or illness incalcitrant to elucidation. It is not preeclampsia. Rather, we know when these bills were submitted, when the bans were debated. We have lists of who voted for and against, the governors who signed or vetoed, the attorney generals who chose to uphold or defend in court. Our abortion bans are not one atom absurd. Everything that has happened to every patient has occurred exactly as someone planned it to occur. If a victim of incest cannot access abortion, it is because the law was written specifically that they could not. Moreover, what would our response be to something that was genuinely absurd? To succumb then to pessimism, to wallow in ennui? In June 2022, none of us awoke to find ourselves cockroaches. Furthermore, we know exactly how to end this. Our laws can be changed, judicial decisions reversed, constitutions amended. The details will vary in differing states. We succeeded in Ohio, though we were also fortunate as our state allows citizen-led ballot initiatives. The pathways in other states are more harrowing, the processes perhaps even years in the making—but they exist; this is not an insolvable problem.

III PHYSICIANS AFTER DOBBS

12 DELIVERY: HOW DO PHYSICIANS SPEAK OUT AFTER DOBBS?

When I first walked into labor and delivery as an intern, I proudly wore my new long white coat as the hard-won trophy from four years of medical school. "Take that off," my chief resident said almost immediately. "Nobody actually wears those. Plus, in obstetrics it will only get stained with blood and coffee."

In public, doctors are always wearing the classic long white coats: in front of a microphone, at the lectern before a legislative committee, holding signs on the steps of a statehouse. All of this belies the white coat's modern frequency in hospitals, where they cloak only an abating cohort of traditionalists; most doctors no longer wear them. On a day-by-day basis, white coats no longer serve any practical use, the former contents of their giant pockets now simply available on your phone. But though we may joke privately about wearing "doctor costumes" in public, we nevertheless still pack and fold them before traveling to advocacy endeavors. Why? Because they match the public's expectation. In the weeks following the Dobbs decision, when the bright lights of the media suddenly shone upon our profession, questions about the public's perception of physicians became increasingly urgent, if not existential.

For several weeks post Dobbs, ob-gyns were in the news constantly, and despite our fears and personal risks, many decided to face this new challenge without hesitation. At one point, it felt like the national news had turned into an OB-GYN Facebook as you could scroll through newspapers and TV programs and see so many of your compatriots. How did we perform in those weeks? Did we act in accordance with how doctors are expected to act?

In public opinion polls, physicians and other healthcare workers remain among the public's most trusted professions. According to the Pew Research Center, 57 percent of US adults say that medical doctors care about the best interests of their patients all or most of the time.[1] About half of Americans surveyed said medical doctors do a good job of providing diagnoses and treatment recommendations. Thus, we have a potentially powerful voice in the public discourse following Dobbs—but are we always able to speak out? Most employers do not have the formal power to stop employees from speaking publicly on issues of policy or public health, so long as they do so independently and not on behalf of their employer and follow their institution's media policies. Likewise, many physicians after Dobbs made their voices heard as private individuals or on behalf of their professional organizations. However, many did not, facing reasonable hesitancy despite an absence of technical prohibition. Power can be formal or informal, with the informal application often the most insidious. What if a young physician, their burgeoning career the fruit of arduous years of training, perhaps with a family to support, spoke out publicly, as was technically permitted, but it was against the implied approval of their department or employer? Later, as the months proceed, they ponder why they are not selected for departmental committees, invited to join research groups, asked to speak at grand rounds. The operating room front desk is curt when scheduling their surgeries; the anesthesiologist after patient intubation is no longer engaging in witty banter.

One of the earliest academic publications examining the impact of new abortion bans was the study mentioned earlier of patients with previable PPROM, published by researchers at the UT Southwestern in October 2022.[2] Because Texas's abortion ban, SB 8, went into effect prior to the Dobbs decision, its medical impacts were the first to be evaluated. The publication sounded alarm through the medical community, social media, and national news organizations, though it did so largely on just its own merit as the university itself never issued the customary press release at the time of publication. Schools usually promote the research of their faculty, but here UT Southwestern was conspicuously silent. Later, when a health reporter from CNN requested an interview with one of the study authors, the university declined to cooperate or allow the researchers to be interviewed in an official capacity, stating the physicians could only do so "as private individuals, independent of their role with the state." Reporters from CNN were never able to conduct the interview; the organization encountered a series of closed doors from hospitals and universities throughout the United States in its attempts to talk to doctors after Dobbs. When CNN reached out to the MD Anderson Cancer Center in Houston to discuss the impact of abortion bans on pregnant cancer patients, its reporters were informed that the center's oncologists were not available for interviews. Ultimately, CNN published an article instead on the suppression of physician voices themselves.[3] As outlined in many anonymous accounts, ob-gyns throughout the country were simultaneously facing an unprecedented crisis and a muzzle.

Years before, after my initial residency graduation, I worked as a general ob-gyn for twelve months prior to a high-risk fellowship. That year entailed a wide range of jobs, including work at a local labor and delivery unit, at a federally funded health center for low-income patients, and at a clinic that provided abortions.

One particular day that year, Operation Save America (OSA) targeted our clinic for a focused day of protest. I cannot tell you exactly what happened outside the building that Friday. The protest plans had been known in advance by supporters monitoring antiabortion message boards, so patients were given warning, our pro-choice escorts mobilized, security and local law enforcement notified, and staff advised to arrive extra early and stay late. Therefore, though I needed to set the alarm clock early and pour extra strong coffee, I never saw anything myself. I arrived and left before and after the protestors, with the inside of the clinic basically quiet given its sturdy walls. With a longer wait before the first patients, the staff and I sat in the break room chatting over bagels and cream cheese, the mood oddly calm despite the growing chaos outside.

Although I did not witness it myself, I later saw a photo of our clinic that Friday engulfed in protesters. Specifically, I saw the photo on the side of my new coffee mug. A few weeks after the OSA protest, our organization gave everyone who worked inside that day a commemorative mug, a picture of our surrounded clinic on one side and "I survived OSA 2004" on the other.

The mug still sits in my office bookshelf, as it has for years, though always with "I survived OSA 2004" facing outward and the photo of the clinic facing only books. If a visitor peruses my shelves, they may not understand the meaning of the text; the direction of the mug thus should render it harmless should that visitor not share my views on abortion. If it was turned around, however, everyone would understand the photograph of protesters surrounding a clinic, even if they do not know the full story. If I know that my visitor supports abortion rights, I take down the mug to show both sides, with me heroically inside a clinic under siege that day. If I do not know the visitor, the picture remains harmlessly facing the books. When talking in my office, I can focus, if I wish, on only MFM, with my year in that clinic sufficiently remote that I have even lost my second-trimester dilation and evacuation (D&E) skills in the intervening decades. Even back in 2004, when asked where I was working, I could select from a range of replies as I had multiple ongoing jobs. If the person asking was supportive of abortion rights, I described working at the clinic on Fridays; if I was unsure, I would just describe the local labor and delivery. These all felt like trivial, minor decisions at the time, just microperformances given to one audience versus another. Prior to Dobbs, how many such microperformances and tiny similar decisions were played out continuously by how many physicians? Decisions that were not brave but also felt, at the time, inconsequential. When we think of the decisions we make in life, we usually think of them on a grand scale. We think of the job search, the surgery, the experimental infusion of antibodies against a virus—not the direction we turn a mug sitting on a shelf. After the Dobbs ruling, however, it is impossible not to look back upon all your prior decisions, regardless of how small, and wonder. How many times have I avoided the subject of abortion with acquaintances or spoken circumferentially in euphemisms? What every doctor had spoken clearly and convincingly with family and friends if prior to Dobbs? What if we had all been just a little braver?

For several weeks after the Dobbs ruling, many OB-GYN physicians spoke out, despite their fears and personal risks. And for so many of us, it was terrifying. But the world needed to know what was occurring after the fall of Roe. Abortion, pregnancy, and even medicine itself are often immersed in confusion and disinformation. As high-risk obstetricians in particular, we bear witness to stories most would never imagine or see. We thus bear the responsibility to advocate as well.

There is a certain irony in the stress felt by high-risk obstetricians when facing television cameras, especially for live events. *High risk* is right there in the name of our field, with our usual lives immersed in emergencies, surgeries, and pending potential tragedies. But when they clip the microphone to your scrubs, the cameras roll, and the reporters ask questions, it's impossible not to feel the tightening of your stomach's knot.

A more specific concern for me is that I have a speech disorder. I speak with a stutter.

I've had a stutter since I can remember, acclimating to it long ago, though I can imagine how strange, if not horrifying, it would be if experienced instead by someone for the first time. Essentially, your brain knows what you want to say, and you try to say it, but instead find yourself standing there doing nothing, or involuntarily repeating the same sound, the pathways between mind and mouth scrambled. It would be as if you were typing on a computer and periodically, randomly, your hands would just freeze, or perhaps you would uncontrollably start pressing one of the buttons over and over.

After copious childhood therapy, I can now navigate most sentences and often whole conversations without stuttering noticeably, though this often requires a vocal sleight of hand. If I steer through a conversation, it is usually because I intentionally dodged triggering words, or I actually did stutter a few times but managed to hide it within a pause or cough. Reading from a script or vocally rehearsing also helps. As a result, I make it safely through most of my academic lectures, though this approach is never foolproof. Basically, any time I talk, my brain is actively, continuously negotiating treacherous waters. When I speak smoothly, it sounds natural, but it is, ironically, artifice; my normal inclination is to stutter, and it is fluency, instead, that constitutes a strained performance. And no matter what I do, there is always a small though present risk of getting totally blocked—hitting a sound I cannot circumvent, the whole vocal stream coming to a standstill like a boat moored upon rocks.

One evening shortly after the Dobbs decision, I arranged to meet a reporter for a national news program to discuss the abortion ban hanging over us. We were scheduled to meet in the evening in the private office of one of my colleagues, the use of which avoided recording during work hours, though the office was also about a forty-minute drive away from where I had been seeing patients that day. As I navigated the increasingly rural roads, running late for the reporter, thoughts of my patients and all my other responsibilities hung over me. The reporter met me at the door, the office staff at the end of their day having let her in before my arrival. She was an efficient, one-person news unit, traversing the country with portable lights, cameras, and microphones, recording events as they occurred. I apologized for running late. In the small bathroom I donned scrubs and a white coat for visual effect, then sat at a table in the consultation room. The shelf behind me was lined with books, a thin microphone wire running under my shirt, the lights and camera set up before me. The first step was straightforward: just start recording, then say my name, location, role, and field—Dr. David Hackney, specialist in maternal fetal medicine, and Ohio Section Chair for the American College of Obstetricians and Gynecologists.

The reporter turned the camera on, giving me the signal to start. I got through my name, then my field, then hit a wall at the *O* in Ohio, vowels being a common trigger for stuttering. I covered it with a cough as if the problem was something stuck in my throat—a commonly used little deception—apologized, and asked to run again. "No worries," she said amicably, resetting the camera. I crashed into the *O* again, my brain refusing to move my mouth, now obviously blocked. The reporter, concerned but also clearly a kind person, again reset the camera. Once again, I started smoothly, then stopped completely at Ohio. Now I was just looking down at the table; the reporter had traveled all the way to our state, was sitting across from me in an empty office in the evening, all to interview me—a physician trapped within a speech disorder. Every time I make a decision to talk or give a lecture or an interview, I do so assuming some risk of getting stuck. At that time after Dobbs, I had given many successful interviews, including live national events—but I always fundamentally knew I was playing with fire, that one day my luck would run out. You cannot gamble forever and not eventually draw a losing hand. Maybe deep inside I had just been in denial of this facticity in my life, that this was all just a dangerous mistake.

After a while, I said, slowly, that it had been a stressful day and I just needed a minute and a glass of water. The reporter told me to take as long as I needed, do what I had to do. The camera was clicked off, the microphone disengaged. I walked down the hall into the office bathroom and closed the door behind me.

When you have a speech disorder, every decision to talk is weighed carefully, balancing the scenario, urgency, audience, and words. But underlying everything is actually an even more fundamental decision, one so basic you can easily forget it is a decision at all: the decision to care in the first place about what others think. I did not choose any of this. I did not choose to have a speech disorder. I did not choose for Roe to be overturned. I did not choose this fight. But we all face facts in our lives, and we all then have to make decisions.

I drank some water from the bathroom sink. Quietly, I made myself say the word *Ohio*, then again and again. *Ohio. Ohio.* I sat back down in the chair; the reporter reconnected the microphone. My name is Dr. David Hackney, I practice maternal fetal medicine in Cleveland, and am the Ohio Section Chair for the American College of Obstetricians and Gynecologists.

13 OATH: HAVE OUR HIPPOCRATIC RESPONSIBILITIES CHANGED AFTER DOBBS?

Other than perhaps the long white coat, little else in the public mind is as closely associated with medicine as the Hippocratic oath. Physicians who support reproductive rights say that abortion bans violate their oaths. Alternatively, physicians who oppose them claim that the Hippocratic oath prohibits abortion. Most often, however, the oath is fashioned into a weapon wielded against doctors by those outside of medicine; our critics use it to accuse us of having somehow broken an ancient bond. In a Pennsylvania senate race, Dr. Oz was accused of violating the oath in his opposition to abortion rights.[1] Alternatively, Indiana's attorney general, who supports abortion bans, accused an ob-gyn of failing to uphold "Hippocratic responsibilities."[2] Often, when pundits use the oath to attack us, it is with some air of sophisticated identification with the ancient Greeks, or a presumption that they have now triumphantly discovered our fatal flaw, trapped us with our own oath to which we are sworn. But do physicians in modern times still actually take the oath? What does the oath say about abortion? And how has our relationship to the oath changed since the Dobbs ruling?

Over two thousand years ago, Hippocrates was born into medicine, the profession at the time centered within familial guilds. His family, the Asclepiad, believed themselves descendants of their namesake, the demigod Aesculapius the Surgeon, and Hippocrates in turn learned medicine directly from his father and grandfather. Later, he made the new, radical assertion that a person could *choose* to become a physician rather than only be destined to be one at birth. He founded the medical school at Kos, whose greatest innovation may have just been that it was, in the first place, a school—an institute where a person could choose to enroll rather than learn only from within one's family. Hippocrates himself did not write the Hippocratic oath. It is instead confusingly named from a large body of writings called the *Hippocratic Corpus*, crafted from multiple authors over many decades at the school that bore his name. However, like the school itself, a critical aspect of the oath was simply the independent decision to take it if one wished.

In 2010's underrated children's movie *Megamind*, two alien babies, in a spoof of Superman's mythology, are rocketed into space from their dying home planets. Upon reaching Earth, one character, Metro Man, coasts through a home's front door into a family's loving arms while the other, Megamind, crashes into a prison for the criminally insane. Both then grow up in the circumstances into which they had been thrown. Metro Man matures into a hero and Megamind a villain, each learning the outward portrayal of their archetype. Then the main character, the criminal Megamind, embarks on a hero's journey. He evolves from comical heel to the city's savior, risking himself in the movie's climax to battle evil, discovering the existence into which he had been thrown not to be his actual chosen essence.

His counterpart, the heroic Metro Man, meanwhile holds down the B or possibly C plot; he is initially raised as a hero in accordance with his powers, upbringing, and masculine jawline. At risk of spoiling an old movie, he is believed to be killed early in the plot, with Megamind having finally succeeded against his archnemesis. Later, however, the movie reveals that Metro Man faked his death intentionally in order to become a recluse. When the main characters eventually find him, he sheepishly concedes that he no longer wants to be a superhero; he has grown weary of saving the city. In an explanatory flashback, we learn that he used his super speed during Megamind's attack to freeze time. He was then finally given the leisure to read books and stroll through a sunny park; he was granted space to think for once, despite the swirling comic book chaos, discovering that he didn't authentically want to perform the superhero role. "I began to realize, despite all of my powers, each and every citizen of Metro had something I didn't, a choice."[3] But Metro Man also had a choice: He chose to fake his death and walk away, quietly learning to play the guitar in his secluded enclave with the movie's A plot churning away out of sight.

The scene is played comically, the reactions of other characters exaggerated, wide-eyed and jaw slackened. But what if we instead chose to consider Metro Man seriously? What if the franchise underwent one of those dark, gritty superhero reboots, something directed by Christopher Nolan or Zack Snyder? In the original movie, Metro Man reveals the truth from inside his hidden lair, while outside the villain Tighten relentlessly assaults the city, slicing entire collapsing buildings with his laser vision, while the cartoon glosses over the fact that in reality he would be slaughtering thousands. The other characters are thus incredulous, refusing to believe Metro Man will not come to their rescue. What if Metro Man again acquiesces, returns to the fight? There is always a Tighten, a Megamind, another monster from which he must save the city—but Metro Man wants to learn the guitar. Does he never then read the book he wants to read, strum the chords he wants to play, fly a kite on that sunny day in the park? Decades later, does he look back with heroic pride or sad regret? If we make decisions according to our abstract moral virtues, then he needs to save the city. If we instead focus on only concrete consequences, adding the total utility of our competing options and then selecting the quantitatively greatest good, he again needs to save the city. If you balance all the guitars and kites and books and sunny days against the human suffering of Tighten's rampage, then Metro Man needs to stop Tighten. Even without having ever taken any formal oath, Metro Man morally, mathematically, ethically, and logically needs to save the city. But he does not want to save the city. He does not want to be Metro Man. He wants to play the guitar.

But can Metro Man not be Metro Man? He changes his name to *Music Man*, though when Tina Fey's character strikes him in anger with his guitar it still shatters apart harmlessly. To paraphrase the ending of *Kill Bill*: Metro Man did not *become* Metro Man; Metro Man was *born* Metro Man. When Metro Man wakes up in the morning, he *is* Metro Man: His clothes are his costume, his powers his powers.

At the height of the COVID pandemic, healthcare workers became engulfed in the vernacular of superheroes: pictures of the nurse with a bright yellow "S" emblazoned across their chest, the physician with a golden lasso and bracers. But though we battled a pandemic killing thousands, we are not superheroes. We were not rocketed as babies to earth, raised by Amazonians on a hidden island, or endowed with a green glowing ring from a dying alien. Nor were we born like Hippocrates into a mystical guild of physicians tracing their lineage back to ancient Greek gods. When we stood in our hospitals on those terrifying days, it was because we intentionally made the decisions that led us there: what to study in high school, which classes to take in college, where to apply, which specialties to enter. In any final analysis, every doctor is a doctor because they have made the choice to be a doctor. When we awoke in the morning, we were humans who made the choice to drive into labor and delivery, the ICU, or the emergency room. In 2020, we were not bulletproof or encased in suits of mechanized armor; rather, we were also susceptible to the virus and could die like anyone else—and early in the pandemic, we began to die.

A report by the *Guardian* and the Kaiser Foundation[4] estimated that 3,600 American healthcare workers died in concert with their duties during the pandemic's first year, a number that included not only physicians and nurses but everyone upon whom hospitals critically rely: patient transporters, unit administrators, the environmental workers who clean the emergency department or ICU rooms. As is sadly common, healthcare worker COVID deaths were sharply disproportionate across economic, racial, and ethnic demographics. The International Council of Nurses estimated that 115,000 healthcare workers died globally in the fight against COVID.[5] For physicians, researchers at Stanford University estimated that 622 American doctors died from the pandemic in the line of duty.[6] Ob-gyns in particular who lost their lives facing the virus included Dr. Luis Caldera-Nieves of Miami, Florida; Dr. Arthur Tayengco of Las Vegas, Nevada; and Dr. Jack Zoller of New Orleans, Louisiana.[7] In October 2020, the death of an OB-GYN resident in Texas, Dr. Adeline Fagan, sent waves of grief through our medical communities.

I myself had COVID severity risk factors, being both overweight and with complex hypertension. On Twitter, I followed the Faces of COVID account, which humanized the pandemic by posting the pictures and stories of those who died, helping prevent our collective collapse into cold statistics. The COVID victims were as diverse as humanity itself, including many that looked like me: larger, bearded men with flannel shirts and hearty smiles. I gained weight from the stress and my closed gym, and then my blood pressure spun dangerously out of control. In the morning, while eating breakfast, I would scroll through Faces of COVID; then on the drive to work I would blast music to suppress the voice in my head telling me I was going to die, that my colleagues and friends in medicine were going to die, that my residents and fellows in training were going to die.

What if one day we didn't want to face COVID, did not want to go into the hospital? The virus was relentlessly assaulting our city, killing thousands. If we make decisions in accordance with our best moral virtues, we needed to drive to the hospital. If we focused instead on only concrete consequences, adding up the total utility of competing options and then engaging in the greatest good, we again needed to go to the hospital. Morally, mathematically, ethically, and logically, we needed to keep working. But what if we didn't want to do so? Are we not then held to an oath?

In the 1990s, on my first day of medical school, I fully anticipated taking the Hippocratic oath. I was the first in my family to enter medicine and thus harbored many inaccurate presumptions. I envisioned the oath as a guiding principle, a compass always pointing north that I could consult in times of ethical uncertainty. It would be my new code, ceremonially handed to me, thereafter superseding whichever other frameworks I had carried in with me. If asked that first day about my current principles, I would have likely ranted about college radio as I had previously been the general manager of my station, Carnegie Mellon's WRCT. I would have espoused upon the economics of the music industry, the noble quest for authenticity achieved by shunning the mass-produced and instead playing the 7″ vinyl with Jawbox covering Tar on one side and Tar covering Jawbox on the other. The University of Chicago Pritzker School of Medicine required an application essay about someone who had influenced you. I wrote mine about the time in high school I met punk legend Ian MacKaye after a Fugazi concert at Pittsburgh's Upstage Lounge. When I nervously asked for his autograph, he declined and instead talked to me kindly about the dangers of celebrity culture and idolization of others above yourself. My resultant essay was an erstwhile treaty on the ethical principles of indie rock, particularly Dischord Records, and how they could be applied to medicine. Everyone said the essay was an awful idea—and the essay was an awful idea; the University of Chicago rejected me without even an interview.

But like most physicians, I did not take the Hippocratic oath in 1996 and never have. In a 2018 survey of American medical schools, no respondent used the original oath, with over half employing instead an idiosyncratic pledge written by the school itself.[8] Like several schools, we recited the Declaration of Geneva as an alternative to the oath. Many institutions now have students write their own oaths to reflect their own values. Some use an oath symbolically called "Hippocratic" but written in modern times.[9] Certainly, many of the principles espoused by the oath, such as patient confidentiality and nonmaleficence, remain bedrocks of modern medical ethics—just not the literal, original oath itself.

Why do doctors no longer take the Hippocratic oath? Among other reasons, it is over 2,000 years old and begins thus: "I swear by Apollo the physician, and Aesculapius the surgeon, likewise Hygenia and Panacea and call all the gods and goddesses to witness, that I will observe and keep this underwritten oath, to the utmost of my power and judgment." The four referenced gods are a family, with Apollo the father of Aesculapius, whose many children included Hygenia and Panacea. These children of Aesculapius then constituted his lineage, the Asclepiad, into which Hippocrates, his father, and his grandfather believed themselves born. Two of Aesculapius's children are also named in the Hippocratic oath: Hygenia, the goddess of cleanliness, and Panacea, the goddess of the universal remedy. While Aesculapius' other children not referenced in the oath slid over the centuries into obscurity, Hygenia and Panacea to his day influence medical thought and semantics: Hygenia is the origin of the word *hygiene*, and a *panacea* symbolizes the certain, perfect solution to an illness or problem. The goddess Panacea would carry in her hands a vial of medicine, the consumption of which could cure any disease; she would wander with it through the ancient land to cure all ills.

The tales of Apollo and Aesculapius entertainingly illuminate our history and symbolism, though as a reflection of the oath's age they were presumed at the time written to be literal. Thus, though its concepts still inform modern ethics, the actual use of the oath faded away decades in the past. This was illustrated in the 1972 oral arguments of *Roe v. Wade* itself when the justices, in concert with usual public expectation, were confused to have not seen any reference to the oath in documents or oral arguments up to that point. The following is an exchange from the court transcripts:

> **Question:** Tell me why you didn't discuss the Hippocratic oath.
>
> **Mrs. Weddington:** Okay.
>
> I guess it was—okay—in part because the Hippocratic oath, we discussed basically the constitutional protection we felt the woman to have. The Hippocratic oath does not pertain to that.
>
> Second, we discuss the fact that the State had not established a compelling State interest. The Hippocratic oath would not really pertain to that. And then we discuss the vagueness jurisdiction.
>
> It seemed to us that the fact that the medical profession at one time had adopted the Hippocratic oath does not weigh upon the fundamental constitutional rights involved. It is a guide for physicians, but the outstanding organizations of the medical profession have in fact adopted a position that says the doctor and the patient should be able to make the decision for themselves in this kind of situation.
>
> **Question:** Of course it's the only definitive statement of ethics of the medical profession. I take it from what you said that you didn't even footnote it because it's old. That's about, really, what you're saying.
>
> **Mrs. Weddington:** Well, I guess it is old, and not that it's out of date, but that it seemed to us that it was not pertinent to the argument we were making.[10]

Although no longer routinely taken by physicians, the oath remains steadfast in the public's imagination, even though its concepts are vague and malleable enough to be crafted by many different speakers to serve many different purposes. Likewise, it is often cited both in support of[11] or opposition to[12] abortion bans. Does the original oath prohibit abortion? This hinges on variable interpretations of the ancient Greek, the debate centering on if the authors opposed abortion writ large or just one specific method—namely, "abortive pessaries," bundles of herbs placed vaginally. These pessaries had a dangerous potential for heavy bleeding and were thus often advised against. The opinion of Hippocrates himself on abortion is unknown as, regardless of how one interprets the ancient Greek, Hippocrates was not the oath's actual author, as previously detailed.

I suspect the reason that so many still presume physicians take the oath is our tendency to believe what we want to be true. The concept of the oath is certainly reassuring. Imagine a patient in an operating room drifting away under anesthesia who finds comfort in the idea of their physicians having all taken an ancient oath, or a populace in a deadly pandemic believing that doctors will remain stationed at their hospitals to face death themselves, an oath preventing them from instead secluding themselves away to learn the guitar.

The public may now reasonably ask what guides medicine's decisions in its absence, and it should be assured that foregoing the Hippocratic oath did not just abandon us into an ethical vacuum. Rather, several modern codes exist, such as the American Medical Association Code of Medical Ethics and guidelines from specific professional organizations—for me, the American College of Obstetricians and Gynecologists—all of which are in addition to our federal, state, and hospital rules and regulations. Medical students also still take oaths of other sorts. Despite never taking the Hippocratic oath, I believe I act ethically and in my patients' interests. Especially in MFM, where we regularly face ethical dilemmas—even more so now under abortion bans. Medical ethics themselves are never static but instead evolve continually with changes in society and medicine, hopefully as part of a process of continued improvement. Another example of evolution is perhaps the Hippocratic oath itself, now consigned to antiquity, but in its time a radical departure from the Asclepiad medical philosophy into which Hippocrates had been born.

How have our codes, oaths, and ethics changed under Dobbs? The American Medical Association, among other organizations, had to update its policies in the wake of abortion bans. The preamble to the code of ethics now states, "In exceptional circumstances of unjust laws, ethical responsibilities should supersede legal duties."[13] A subsequent perspective on the change entitled "Professional Civil Disobedience—Medical-Society Responsibilities After Dobbs" was published in the *New England Journal of Medicine*.[14] In the opinion piece, the bioethicist Dr. Mathew Wynia outlines the moral case for physicians to violate the law if to do otherwise would cause patient harm, drawing parallels to other historical examples such as those in the Soviet Union and apartheid South Africa. But is this now our binding moral code after Dobbs? If faced with such a choice, are doctors now ethically required to disobey at all other costs? Furthermore, this changed code is not the oath I had taken as a medical student, when the prospect of future criminal jeopardy would have been viewed as absurd. As our codes, oaths, and risks all change continuously with time, so must each individual always recalculate their own positioning.

A wanderer gazes from atop a hillside into a valley below and sees monsters moving among the villagers from house to house. Do they descend into the valley to help? Once there, which homes do they rescue? Presuming the valley will always have houses and monsters, when then do they choose to leave? It is natural to group all three questions into one, for if you do not descend, choose some path, and then choose to remain, then no houses are ultimately rescued. But each of the questions also holds its own calculus, related to the others but not identical.

My wife and I met as medical students and trained together as residents. Although she knew early on that she wanted to enter pediatrics, she had not initially selected children's cancer specifically. Originally, she was fascinated by childhood kidney diseases, preparing to enter fellowship in pediatric nephrology. But she kept gazing instead into that other valley, with its distressed families and formidable monsters. We together surveyed those dark forests, seeing with clear eyes exactly what they held.

Once when we were early in our careers, just shortly out of training, we were on a group tour of an archeological site. The afternoon started with a social gathering with food and drinks in an outdoor patio before we all strolled out with the guide. Conversing with an older couple, my wife discovered that by coincidence he too had once been a pediatric oncologist, later leaving cancer to work in a general outpatient office instead. My wife, a junior in the same field looking down her own career road, was naturally curious as to why he had left his. So, under the bright sun and with a second glass of red wine, he told her his story.

When he was first training in the 1970s, childhood cancer was far more harrowing than it is even now, with few effective therapies in existence and survival rates far lower than with modern treatments. Thus, early in his career, many of the children he cared for suffered and died—but then, slowly, inch by painful, tragic inch, the field advanced. New chemotherapies emerged; scientists progressively found cures; more children were rescued to instead live into adulthood. A decade later, one would need not be an optimist to believe the future bright, to believe that, although death would never be completely vanquished, there would be only continued progress in subsequent years. Then one of the patients he had successfully treated, one of his precious, heartwarming triumphs in the often-bleak battle against childhood cancer, returned suddenly with overwhelming infection and a disastrously low white blood cell count. The child died shortly thereafter of sepsis. Then another child presented with the same mysterious illness: the plummeting white blood cell count, the unstoppable infections. Later scientists would identify the new virus, HIV; though originally unknown at that time, it had infiltrated the blood supply. Because the children he treated often required many transfusions over many years, an unquantified though likely sizable number were now infected, and one by one they returned to the hospital, with no available therapies as even the most basic antiretroviral medications were still years away in the future. These were the children he had saved, the children given the new chemotherapeutic agents, the newest radiation treatments. These were the children who were supposed to have ridden out of the hospital on white horses into the sunset to live happy lives but who were now lying in beds again with IVs and blood draws, fighting an enemy that could not be defeated, against which existed no curative treatments, no curative hope.

As a student in the 1970s, he had gazed into pediatric oncology and saw the monsters there, roaming mostly freely at the time as there existed few therapeutic weapons against them. Against these odds, he freely chose to descend into the valley, where he then lived for years, often failing but always studying the monsters, learning how they moved and when they struck. He fashioned new weapons, others choosing to join him as well, and then together they rescued those previously lost. But one day a new monster arrived, one nobody had seen before, a monster against which he had no weapons—not even initially a basic understanding of its movements and methods. Against this monster he would be helpless, with nothing to do but watch from among the trees as it moved from house to house.

But perhaps more importantly, this was not the monster he had chosen to face; it was not roaming the valley years before when he had surveyed as a student. This was a monster he now had to decide if he should fight, with him always free to leave instead. Never had he made to Greek deities an oath to remain forever in this valley. So, he sadly packed away his backpack and ascended. Later, as a general pediatrician, he spent his days with vaccinations, earaches, and runny noses, signing paper forms for middle school sport participation; as parents know, all this is critically important and also sometimes not without its own monsters, just not the monsters roaming the valley he had left. And now here he was, decades later, his hair thick grey, the day bright, accidentally spilling some of his wine as he spoke. Later we toured the site, the guide explaining how the structures were built with heavy stones, those in the past diligent despite the limited tools of their time. The pediatrician smiled peacefully as we moved together along the path, two small, dark red stains on his white shirt.

When my classmates and I surveyed medicine as college students and made the choice to enter, we also were not then making the decision to face COVID years later in 2020. But then a new monster roared upon us, and we all had to decide again. When we surveyed obstetrics as medical students, we also were not making the decision to one day face criminal jeopardy, but then in 2022 we all had to make choices again. In many ways, it felt unjust for our field to face the fallout of Dobbs so soon after having endured the COVID pandemic, but politicians who now aim legislative powers against us should know they face physicians who have just stood together arm in arm against death.

When the teachers at Hippocrates's school were writing their oath, the goddess Panacea and her cup of medicine were not only presumed factual but held as an ideal toward which physicians should strive. But now we no longer believe in Panacea herself or magical, all-curing medications. Our use of the concept has flipped completely, references to a treatment being a panacea now ironic if not outright derisive, with one who believes something a panacea a fool. But it is hard sometimes not to wish for the Hippocratic oath as I had imagined it to exist before that first day of medical school, now that we often face situations in which we don't know what to do. If we could just offer an oath in return for some specific wisdom that had weathered millennia, then not only would it show us where to go, but we would be bound to follow it above all other concerns. We would not have to make the difficult decisions we face after Dobbs. But no Greek deities are coming to help us. There is no Panacea. It is just us.

14 RESPONSIBILITY: WHERE DO A PHYSICIAN'S OBLIGATIONS END?

In June 2022, I was entirely unprepared for our state's abortion ban. In retrospect, this should not have been the case. An anonymous source had leaked the Dobbs decision weeks in advance. Our attorney general publicly intended to request the injunction against our ban be lifted once the decision was issued. As a result, before June, as a medical professional in a leadership position, I should have had plans in place, protocols at the ready. I should have read and reread the language of our ban ahead of the injunction falling. Instead, that night in my kitchen, I opened my laptop, searched for, and then began to read the law to which I was already subject. In the weeks that followed, in multiple conversations with multiple colleagues, I discovered that everyone had been in the same boat. Physicians in leadership positions everywhere that night also searched for and read the law's text, sending nervous emails with detailed questions to their lawyers. Perhaps we thought the leaked opinion was not true or that protections would not fall immediately after it was issued or that there still would have been some buffer during which to prepare. But in retrospect, I should have been prepared.

Under an abortion ban, what are the responsibilities of medical leaders? Normally during times of crisis, we provide guidance to physicians. During the COVID pandemic, we crafted protocols and delineated best medical practices. But the questions that arose under abortion bans were legal rather than medical. The responsibility for this guidance should then fall upon those who wrote the laws or are in positions to enforce them. However, political leaders in many states refuse this responsibility.

As part of their role, physicians take on the responsibility for their patients' care, feeling accountable for medical decisions. Years ago, when I was packing to move to Cleveland, I happened to open a box my wife had packed and labeled "Miscellaneous." I forget what I was looking for, but inside, among keepsakes and mementos, was a stack of order of service programs, the pamphlets handed to you by ushers as you enter a funeral. They usually feature a picture of the deceased from earlier, happier times, then the dates of birth and death, a brief description of their life, and finally an order of service outlining the ceremony about to occur. The stack I held was from the funerals my wife had attended. On each pamphlet, the face of a child or teenager smiled back. The dates between birth and death were all too close, sometimes within the same decade. The descriptions of life were short, and the stack of programs held in my hand was not thin. I returned the papers to the box, then closed it with tape.

One day years later, I came home to find a beautiful card hanging by a magnet on our refrigerator door among the drawings from our kids and memos to ourselves. I knew what it likely was before reading it; it was addressed to my wife from the mother of a patient, previously with cancer and now in remission, a young boy. The letter was what someone would write to a superhero who with elastic arms saved your child from a speeding train, a child for whom an entire adolescence, adulthood, and even old age now stretched in front of them. It was beautiful, heartfelt, and, justifiably, neither the first nor last letter of its type to appear in our kitchen. The card brought my wife joy, though as usual she demurred being self-congratulatory when we spoke later that evening. She minimized her contributions, doubted if everything written in it were really true. When I playfully protested, she proceeded to tell me the child's story.

It was the little boy's parents who first noticed something amiss, bringing him to the general pediatrician who ordered blood work and imaging. A radiologist responsible for evaluating the scan identified the mass that the surgeon subsequently removed. The pathologist was then responsible for the correct diagnosis under a microscope. At this point, the oncologist, my wife, was consulted, and she selected chemotherapy on the basis of prior clinical trials for which she had not been personally responsible. The drugs themselves were manufactured in a facility hundreds of miles away. The hospital pharmacist prepared the medications, which then infused into the child through an IV placed by a skilled pediatric nurse. After many rounds of chemotherapy, an imaging study was repeated, then interpreted again by the radiologist, confirming that the tumor remained in remission. My wife tells the mother the good news, and a few days later a card appears in our kitchen.

I know this story trivializing her role is incomplete, that she is a skilled physician with a warm bedside manner who guided this mother and son through a terrifying, almost unimaginable ordeal. She listened carefully as they had questions, monitored the child closely after chemotherapy—but as I assemble the case on her behalf, she stops me to tell another story of another patient, a story that does not end with a card hanging on our refrigerator.

Maybe this child's primary doctor at first misattributed their symptoms to a common cold. Then perhaps the radiologist does not see the mass, or it was initially too subtle. Later in the operating room, the surgeon cannot fully remove the tumor as portions are entangled within blood vessels or vital organs. The optimal chemotherapy does not yet exist, not yet invented by the scientists in the laboratory. Other infusions are trialed, then halted when side effects arise. My wife reads through papers, racking her brain for therapies, talks to other experts, reviews with surgeons, contemplates radiation. Then one day she walks into a stately house of worship where under an arched entryway the usher hands her a beautiful square of heavy white paper adorned with the picture of a happy child. What does she say to herself standing in that doorway, holding the paper, songs about rainbows playing through the speakers? How do we view responsibility in that moment? What are the stories we tell ourselves when we fail? Do we say that it was out of our control, that it was not specifically our fault?

In medicine, physicians try to see differently the outcomes over which we do or do not have control. We don't control the birth defect arising randomly without risk factors, the stray bullet, or the disease emerging anew in a healthy patient. We may have control over an operation, optimal medication dosage, or reading the ultrasound's grey-and-white swirl of shadows. But as physicians, into which category would we place a new law, or electoral changes impacting healthcare? Are they lumped with events outside our control? Natural disasters or random genetic mutations? Or are these also our responsibility?

Consider, as an example, Texas right now. Who is responsible for providing guidance to physicians in questions of abortion? The state attorney general? The Texas Supreme Court? The Texas Medical Board? Physicians in their own judgement?

When Kate Cox was pregnant in Texas, the professional opinion of her obstetrician, Dr. Damla Karsan, was that abortion was her best medical course. Her pregnancy was complicated by *trisomy 18*, a severe genetic condition in which there are three copies of chromosome 18 instead of the usual two. The predominance of pregnancies with trisomy 18 result in stillbirth or early neonatal death, with the uncommon survivors having numerous medical problems, including difficulties breathing and eating, multiple congenital anomalies, and severe intellectual disability. Given the obstetric risks, including for Cox her history of a prior cesarean delivery, a D&E was recommended by her physician. From within the limitations of just what is known publicly, I would personally agree. A district court judge agreed as well, issuing a temporary restraining order to allow the abortion to proceed. However, the Texas attorney general, an individual with no medical training or expertise, disagreed, issuing an open letter to the three involved hospitals that outlined potential first-degree felony prosecutions. The case then moved to the Texas Supreme Court, which ruled against Cox.

But had Dr. Karsan's professional assessment not been that her patient met the law's medical requirements? Was this not sufficient? The ruling stated: "Dr. Karsan asserted that she has a 'good faith belief' that Ms. Cox meets the exception's requirements. Certainly, a doctor cannot exercise 'reasonable medical judgment' if she does not hold her judgment in good faith. But the statute requires that judgment be a 'reasonable medical' judgment, and Dr. Karsan has not asserted that her 'good faith belief' about Ms. Cox's condition meets that standard."[1]

As a layperson, this explanation is baffling. Even more perplexing is that the court additionally asserts the responsibility of physicians for their own medical judgment while at the same time questioning and disregarding the medical judgement of Dr. Kasan: "A woman who meets the medical-necessity exception need not seek a court order to obtain an abortion. Under the law, it is a doctor who must decide that a woman is suffering from a life-threatening condition during a pregnancy, raising the necessity for an abortion to save her life or to prevent impairment of a major bodily function. The law leaves to physicians—not judges—both the discretion and the responsibility to exercise their reasonable medical judgment, given the unique facts and circumstances of each patient."[2]

Essentially, here someone is attempting to thread an impossibly thin needle by not formally disagreeing with the physician's medical judgment—in fact, holding up physician judgment as primary—while at the same time explaining why Dr. Kasan's best medical judgment is still insufficient for Cox to actually receive care.

The Texas Supreme Court ruling furthermore stated that responsibility for additional guidance falls upon the Texas Medical Board: "The courts cannot go further by entering into the medical-judgment arena. The Texas Medical Board, however, can do more to provide guidance in response to any confusion that currently prevails."[3] It then states that the medical board could "assess various hypothetical circumstances, provide best practices, identify red lines, and the like."

After the Texas Supreme Court ruling, Molly Duane, the lawyer representing Cox, told *The New York Times*: "Essentially, what we have is that no one will take responsibility. The court isn't taking responsibility. The medical board isn't taking responsibility."[4]

The Texas Medical Board did later release clarifying rules in response to the Texas Supreme Court, though they mainly just reiterated definitions for terms such as *abortion*, *ectopic pregnancy*, and *medical emergency* and how to administratively document the abortion indications. Absent was specific medical guidance or the "hypothetical circumstances, best practices, and red lines" suggested by the court. The board also emphasized, accurately, that the critical questions of civil and criminal liabilities were not within their responsibilities: "The rule also explains the limitation of any Board decision and that possible criminal or civil action under the law is separate and independent of any Board decision."[5] In other words, even if the board had provided meticulous guidance detailing exact diagnoses or laboratory values, it could only do so within the purview of the board pertaining to issues such as disciplinary actions and licensure. Physicians would have no formal protections from civil and criminal risk. Instead, physicians are repetitively told to use their own best judgement, but without guarantees that their judgement will not one day be second-guessed. Doctors right now bear the entirety of responsibility.

To make matters worse, these bans are impacting obstetrics during a time when our country has some of the worst pregnancy outcomes in the industrialized world. America's preterm birth rate in 2022 was 10.4 percent, earning a D+ grade from the March of Dimes. By contrast, the preterm birth rate in Canada, our neighbor to the north, was most recently 8.3 percent.[6] America's 2022 *infant mortality rate*, defined as the number of infant deaths in the first year of life, was 5.4 per 1,000 births, compared to 4 per 1,000 in Canada. Although this difference may not appear large at first, imagine our millions of annual births and then about one additional child not dying per one thousand born. Our maternal mortality rate was 22.3 deaths per 100,000. All these statistics are also tragically and disproportionately increased for minoritized populations.

How will abortion bans impact national pregnancy outcomes? At the time of writing, we are still largely awaiting epidemiological data as public health records take time to be collected and analyzed. Concern also exists about potential state interference with data reporting, even if just in delays or limitations in what is made public. Case in point: The Maternal Mortality and Morbidity Review Committee (MMMRC) of the Texas Department of State Health Services (DSHS) is legally responsible for releasing a biannual report on maternal deaths. The prior report had been due on September 1, 2022. As Texas's ban predated the Dobbs decision, this would have thus been one of the first public health reports from a state without abortion access. The release also would have occurred before voters went to the polls in November for midterm elections. However, September 2022 came and went with no report, despite a clear legal responsibility. Instead, a plan was announced for the data to be released the following summer. On November 3, the Society for Maternal-Fetal Medicine and the Democracy Forward organization sent a public letter to the Texas DSHS demanding the maternity data, with a plan to pursue legal action in the event of continued noncompliance. It finally then was released on December 16—before the summer, but well after the November elections.

When people play politics with public health records, they should always remember what this data truly represents. Within the panoply of government reports, this is not an index of housing prices or the prospectus of pension funds, but rather the lives of people living in the state. Maternal mortality records specifically are reports of the pregnant patients who have died, and their review not only assists in the care of future patients but also fulfills a responsibility to honor loss.

In addition to maternal mortality, will future data show an impact of abortion bans on preterm birth and infant mortality? The causes of preterm birth are multifactorial, and any population health outcome, like many societal measures, also can be unpredictable. Thus we caution being cavalier in projecting the future. However, abortion bans could contribute to our rates of preterm birth and infant mortality through multiple pathways. Many states right now have no exceptions for fetal congenital and genetic anomalies, which will inevitably contribute to infant mortality. In addition, patients who have conceived in poor health, with conditions such as diabetes, kidney disease, or heart disease, also can no longer access abortion. Alternatively, most patients seeking abortion care are otherwise in good health, and the impact of bans upon the total number of annual abortions so far has not been straightforward, so it is possible that an impact on the overall preterm birth rate may not ultimately manifest in the data.

Over the years, our rates of preterm birth and infant mortality have also remained frustratingly intractable. When I arrived in Cleveland in 2012, Ohio's preterm birth rate was 10.5 percent. Hundreds if not thousands of individuals across the state worked diligently in the intervening decade to improve our obstetric outcomes, yet in 2022 our preterm birth rate was essentially unchanged—if not worsened, at 10.8 percent.

As a high-risk obstetrician, what can I do to prevent preterm birth? If we look only at the administration of a medication or performance of a procedure, we do not have interventions that would prevent the majority of preterm births. A surgery called a *cervical cerclage*, performed upon patients who both have had a prior preterm birth and now have a short cervical length in their current pregnancy, is the intervention with the most solid evidence of benefit from randomized controlled trials. In this context, physicians will prevent roughly one preterm birth for about every eight cerclages they perform, a reasonable balance despite cerclage being a surgical procedure that carries some risks. However, only a fraction of patients who ultimately deliver prematurely are also the exact ones who benefit from a cerclage. Thus, as a broad measure, cerclage would not make a huge impact on preterm birth even if optimally deployed.

What other medical interventions prevent preterm birth? A full exploration would constitute a large textbook chapter, though a reasonable summary is that there exists no pharmacologic silver bullet. Various medications aimed at stopping uterine contractions, called *tocolytics*, have been studied, though none clearly improve pregnancy outcomes. Thus, it is my own practice not to use tocolytics at all. Injections of progesterone were debated and trialed for decades but are now no longer FDA approved or commercially available in the United States due to unclear efficacy. A subset of patients with a short cervix may benefit from vaginal progesterone. Tobacco cessation improves outcomes among patients who smoke. But there ultimately exists no pharmacologic panacea for preterm birth.

What then are the responsibilities of physicians to prevent preterm birth? Is it just to perform a cervical cerclage or prescribe medications? There are many ways to change health outcomes beyond surgery or pharmacologic administrations. The rates of preterm birth within a population, for example, correlate strongly with emotional stress, education, poverty, violence, neighborhood characteristics, and exposure to racism. If we truly want to decrease preterm birth, we would be best served to start by improving our patients' overall lives: help them transcend poverty, reduce stressors, acknowledge racism, enhance safety.

If I made of list of all possible actions, then ranked them by how closely the public associates them with being a physician, what would be their order? At the top would probably be surgery: standing in an operating room adorned in sterile scrubs. Next perhaps would be examining patients, performing radiographic studies, ordering labs, prescribing medications. But where in this ranking would one place a phone call to a congressional office, an interview for the local paper, casting a ballot on Election Day?

Once this ordered list is constructed, where within it would physicians demarcate their responsibilities? Years ago, as a trainee, I would have probably drawn a sharp line at about the list's middle. Someone can also answer this question formally, contractually as an employee or administratively in a job description. In medicine, we have structured delineations of privileges and duties. But what if this question is only answered in the context of the goal of improving our patients' health? Do physicians, for example, have a responsibility to help our patients vote? In a democracy, our leaders disproportionately focus attention and resources upon populations that vote. If all the patients I saw in my office voted in every election, regardless of which candidate they selected, their lives and thus their health would likely improve. Physicians are thus increasingly recognizing voting as a public health goal, with many doctors now incorporating questions about voter registration into their routine inquiries along with seatbelt use or smoking. In 2022, the American Medical Association formally adopted a resolution acknowledging voting as a social determinant of health.

If we draw any line in this list of activities to demarcate our responsibility, the line will be artificial; it will reflect a construct of ourselves as our profession versus us as fully integrated members of the world. In short, there is no line. It is all our responsibility.

15 CARE: CHALLENGES WITH CONTINUING CARE

Perhaps the greatest practical question facing ob-gyns right now is that of working in restrictive states. Where does a resident or fellow move after graduation? Should physicians in states with abortion bans leave? If we do leave, what then happens to our patients and colleagues?

Fundamentally, doctors always want to provide care. During the COVID pandemic, for example, physicians faced byzantine regulations that altered every aspect of our job. We shaved our beards. We stopped wearing ties. We cut our own hair. We diligently covered in masks and entered hospitals through lines awaiting temperature monitoring. If we happened one day to glance at ourselves in the window, we would see someone who appeared far different than they had a few months earlier, but we would still see a doctor providing care. Our core remained fundamentally intact, wholly unencumbered by sartorial changes. The need for care, if anything, grew dramatically during that time. In contrast, life for many ob-gyns in states with abortion bans returned otherwise to normal after the pandemic. An obstetrician in Georgia right now can grow a long beard, wear a tie if they wish, and walk freely through the entrance of their hospital. But they may not be able to provide needed care for their patients—and doctors provide care.

On the day Dobbs was released and bans fell down upon us, I and many Ohio colleagues believed there was nothing we could do, that the future now held no exits. We no longer had the protections of Roe, our legislative bodies were cynically gerrymandered, and the governor, attorney general, and Supreme Court all opposed abortion rights. I was a division chief overseeing my group of high-risk specialists, many of whom I had recruited to Cleveland over the years. In the United States right now are far fewer maternal fetal specialists than are needed to meet hospital needs. Thus, intense competition exists between departments in their hiring and retention. As a division chief, you know that what truly underlies physician recruitment is not your own metrics of leadership or administrative success but the needs of the patients you serve. If I do or do not successfully retain maternal fetal specialists, then our patients with high-risk pregnancies do or do not have access to care.

Shortly after our criminal bans, outside obstetricians still sitting comfortably in permissive states began openly texting our faculty, saying we should leave to join them. Superficially, it smacked of benevolence and concern: There was now nothing to be done here, and if my colleagues stayed, they would only face tragedy and jeopardy. But barely under that surface lay recruitment opportunism. Suddenly, in that already dark moment, we were under attack from not only our state legislature but also members of our own field.

I must pause here to acknowledge the role of privilege in decisions to move out of restrictive states, both when we have the power to leave and when we have the safety to stay. Many people cannot easily relocate secondary to family, economic, or geographic bonds. Alternatively, others may choose to leave due to threats I do not myself encounter in my demographic category. In addition, though the field of maternal fetal medicine is certainly impacted by bans, the predominance of our day-to-day work does not involve abortion, and thus our scenario differs from that of colleagues dedicated entirely to the field of family planning.

But if otherwise freely given the choice, why would we stay in Ohio after our ban? The law appeared at that time ineluctable, our options anemic, our threats real, the future bleak. Doctors always want to do something rather than nothing. We want to operate, intervene, make everything better. We never want our options to be constrained, to be unable to provide care. So much of our preceding education through high school, college, and even medical school entailed waiting frustratingly to do something other than just read books, candy stripe, shadow in offices.

In high school, I volunteered at our local hospital, Passavant, in the northern Pittsburgh suburbs. I somehow had envisioned myself standing in operating rooms or striding through wards elbow to elbow with doctors and nurses. Instead, I discovered that new volunteers in the late 1980s had to serve one hundred hours in the café prior to any greater responsibilities. The small café sat at the hospital entrance, serving the usual coffee, pie, hamburgers, and other foods simple enough to be prepared by teenagers with no particular training. It was brightly lit with long, white linoleum counters and booths. In retrospect, having some screening process for volunteers prior to allowing direct patient contact was reasonable, though at the time one hundred hours mixing shakes and grilling burgers made for a lot of shakes and burgers. On my first day, I met one of the other teens. His long mullet and single pierced ear were not unusual for the time, though they contrasted nonetheless with his bright striped shirt and presumed dreams of medical school acceptance.

"What are you here for?" he asked in a hushed tone, leaning forward, though when I responded with only perplexity, he straightened and continued, louder, now with a hint of pride: "I slashed my neighbor's tires. I do not regret a thing. He was an asshole and had it coming."

"I . . . want to be a doctor?" I stuttered.

After a brief confusion, I discovered that the other teens were juvenile offenders fulfilling mandated community service. It was a blast. We were given meal vouchers for the cafeteria but told not to eat the food from the café itself. However, we found that one volunteer could look out while others made a burger or shake. Never me, of course. The back of the café also connected with the back of the gift shop, which, as it was 1988, carried *Metal Edge Magazine*, a vital resource for adolescents. Theoretically, of course, someone could slip through the back into the gift shop to snag a copy unseen, after which, in the café's slower hours, we could peruse page after page of permed and spandexed guitarists with billowing chest hair.

The busy times around meals, however, were stressful. Unlike any normal restaurant, I am certain none of the customers wanted to be there at all. Nobody was ever just out and about in the suburbs of Wexford, developed a hankering for hot dogs, and elected to patronize the hospital café. These were patients' loved ones, who, no matter how delectably I grilled that burger, would rather be anywhere else. Few smiled; most looked upset. Once I messed up a woman's order; I do not recall how. But when I served the plate, she just burst into tears right there at the linoleum counter, her tears not just sad but furious—not just furious, but furious at me. I stood there stupidly in my red-and-white striped shirt. I presume now that she was experiencing some terrible event, maybe an impending family death, and had just been holding together until I broke the camel's back. The middle-aged manager came over, fixed the order, and waived the charge. "He's just a kid," she said, gesturing toward me with her hand. "He's a volunteer, he makes mistakes." The red-eyed woman quietly ate her food, focusing straight ahead. There were few other customers, so I paced awkwardly behind the counter, avoiding eye contact. A few years later, I put one hundred hours of hospital volunteering on my college applications. Technically, it was completely true; I had certainly spent one hundred hours as a volunteer in a hospital. However, I presumed—to my frustration—that I had learned nothing about medicine at all, had provided no care, had only poured coffee for a sobbing woman holding a somehow incorrect sandwich.

While working that grill, I had wanted desperately to do something, anything that was "medical" in nature, but I believed instead that I was doing nothing. But sometimes as a physician, there are still times when nothing "medical" can be done, even now as a highly trained subspecialist rather than a pimply adolescent. Often we make a horrible diagnosis on fetal ultrasound that consists, fundamentally, of something not being seen that should, a nothingness where instead something should exist. An organ is missing, maybe a limb, maybe even the brain. There is a hole where there should not be a hole. Sometimes a future pediatric surgeon can repair it, or maybe, like a single absent kidney, one will be fine without it—but fundamentally, at that moment there really is nothing medical to do. How many times in my career have my patient recommendations been, if stripped down to their coldest factual core, nothing? Doctors, as a whole, abhor nothing. We avoid talking about nothing, thinking about nothing. All four years of medical school were focused on the *somethings*. Some treatment, some medication, some surgery. I don't recall ever instead having a lecture about nothing—but years later, you complete your training, enter the real world, and suddenly one day there in your office is *nothing*, gazing back at you. Many of medicine's historical mistakes arise from our failing to accept nothing. It is our refusal to accept nothing, for example, that leads us over and over to administer treatments not yet vetted by randomized trials. But our aversion to nothing is also deeply human, nothing being that from which we first arise, then what we define ourselves by making decisions against. Nothing is often the most agonizing choice, which later feels like it was never really a choice at all.

For many obstetricians in states with criminal bans, the future appears desolate. In all states, abortion rights enjoy pluralities of support, though only a few states allow citizen-initiated ballot measures. How long may it be in those states until rights are restored? The wait until a federal remedy is indeterminate; changes may be years away.

Thus, in many states, obstetricians are beginning to leave. Idaho physicians face what are among the most daunting legal jeopardies and in turn are absconding in droves. According to a 2024 report by the Idaho Physician Well-Being Action Collaborative, even before Dobbs the state had only 227 obstetricians.[1] However, after Idaho adopted bans without essentially any exceptions, that number toppled downward to 176. Only two obstetricians have started practicing in Idaho since Dobbs, and 22 percent, almost one in four, have left. Under this disintegration, two labor and delivery units have closed, and with no foreseeable relief, it is unclear when the exodus may taper.

When examining the multitudes leaving restrictive states, we should not lose sight of how difficult it is to move. Laws don't simply change and then the next day everyone packs up boxes. Perhaps you have laid roots in your community, or even just have a robust network of friends. Perhaps your kids are in school, or you just have a favorite corner bar or record shop. None of these details even account for the barriers specific to relocating physicians: state licensure, hospital privileges, insurance networks, referral bases. Imagine all this, and then imagine 22 percent of the obstetricians in Idaho still leaving.

But is there nothing to do for those who choose to stay in restrictive states? As a high school student in the café, I was frustrated, believing my time to be noncontributory—but in actuality, I was still providing care, albeit only the care I was able to provide in that time and situation. Although I could not see it back then, I now recognize those customers as the people you see in medicine all the time: loved ones and patients wanting to be anywhere other than a hospital. The woman whose order I bungled had just wanted a moment of peace at a linoleum counter. Likewise, medicine itself cannot always provide curative therapies. How often back in 1988 had the physicians upstairs, unbeknownst to me on the first floor below, been unable to offer any treatments or hope, but later that day, when the family shuffled to my counter, I was at least able to mix two scoops of vanilla ice cream into a tall glass of root beer and serve it with a striped red straw?

Physicians in restrictive states right now do all the things they are able to do in the situation they are in; they provide all the care they are able to provide. Since Dobbs, many of our most powerful voices have emanated from doctors under bans who have chosen to stay. Rather than face nothingness, they have argued with legislators behind closed doors, served as plaintiffs in litigation, spoken on national stages with crystalline moral clarity. They have helped patients escape. And they have provided care. It may not always be the care they want to provide, should have been legally able to provide, the care that would have best served their patients. But they screen for cancers, provide contraception, treat postpartum depression, and manage infertility. And in every restrictive state, there are thousands upon thousands of patients who need care. Patients need care in Arkansas, in Mississippi, in the Dakotas and Nebraska.

As a number of units close, most US counties now no longer contain a hospital with a labor and delivery unit. However, there may still exist an obstetric provider within the county—for example, an outpatient office where patients can at least receive prenatal care even if they ultimately deliver in the next county over. If a county lacks any provider, contains not a solitary office where pregnant patients can see a physician or midwife, then it is referred to as an *obstetric desert*. The March of Dimes recently released a comprehensive report titled *Nowhere to Go: Maternity Care Deserts Across the US*.[2] The report identified 1,104 such deserts, accounting for 35.1 percent of all US counties. Within these deserts resided 2.3 million pregnancy-capable individuals, who in turn deliver over 150,000 babies annually. The patient risks entailed by such deserts are formidable. If the nearest labor and delivery unit is an hour away, then a patient risks having to travel in the throes of preterm labor, pain, bleeding, or other emergencies. But if someone must also drive an hour for *any* basic obstetric visit or ultrasound, then they might not even access prenatal care at all.

The future likely entails worsening deserts in restrictive states as more obstetricians leave, further risking the patients left behind. But though this outcome is probable, it is also not an inevitability; ultimately, physicians themselves choose where to practice, when to leave, where to go. Leaving may be reasonable, it may be the most prudent decision—but it is a choice. If deserts grow in restrictive states, it is because we have made the decisions to leave. Physician exoduses have layers of responsible parties, including legislators, state attorney generals, and hospital and community support, but in the end, it is the individuals themselves who make the choice to stay or go.

Imagine that a new patient presents to her obstetrician's office for prenatal care. Her family and medical history are uncomplicated, she takes no medications, feels well, and has a normal ultrasound. Then as weeks unfold, her doctor sees her in the clinic, weighs her on the scale, records the blood pressure, measures her expanding abdomen. Her genetic screen is risk reducing, her fetus structurally typical on ultrasound. She does not encounter listeria or cytomegalovirus or toxoplasmosis, does not experience bleeding or preeclampsia; her membranes remain intact until term. At visits, the physician provides guidance and reviews symptoms, makes plans for the normal labor that eventually occurs without complications. In the hospital, the delivery is joyous, the postpartum recovery routine.

For the patient, that birth may be among life's most momentous events—but how is this care viewed instead through medicine's colder, most objective lens? Uncomplicated: The insurer will reimburse the delivery at the lowest rate. Routine: No colleagues will later complement the doctor in the break room. The pregnancy will not be written into scholarly journals or presented at academic meetings. This will not be a story the physician tells legislators one day behind a lectern. The patient will never relay their experience to reporters on news programs. Even that same night with the doctor back at home eating takeout from foil bins, they will monosyllabically respond "fine" when asked about their day.

But this obstetrician lives in a state with restrictive laws, worsening year over year, progressively encroaching upon a range of reproductive care. Each legislative session, they cannot believe the new laws being introduced. Each day in the office, they see the downstream impacts these laws have on their patients. They drive to the statehouse to testify before legislators, who later choose to believe other purported experts instead. They write op-eds in the local paper, unsure if they are read. In each election, they cast ballots that are then overwhelmed by the votes of others. They talk at night with their partner about leaving.

In this scenario, that afternoon's medically routine delivery becomes, in many ways, a blistering act of defiance. Defiance against forces pushing them away from their state and into safer cities on the coasts, defiance against pessimism and nihilism, against the specter of criminal jeopardy and agonizing ethical decisions. It is also the dedication to still providing the care one can provide, because regardless of regulations and laws, there are always patients who need care.

So they freely decide to stay and provide care. Over the years, many of their colleagues do not. Friends from medical school urge them to leave for unrestrictive states, using arguments that are logical, rational, and sensible. But we are never required to make decisions that are logical, rational, or sensible. If we always made the most sensible choices, then we would just go through life being sensible. It is our irrational decisions that are the most human, *because* they are irrational.

If I could freely choose any historical period in which to practice medicine, I would choose to be a doctor right now. Over the last years, healthcare has faced unprecedented turmoil from restrictive laws, disinformation campaigns, and a viral pandemic that killed many of us. I would not wish for these to exist, though if they are to occur, I would rather be here than in some clement future. And if I had to choose colleagues to be here with, I would choose my friends and colleagues right now all around the country.

On the day of the Dobbs decision, obstetricians in Ohio had to decide to stay or leave. Other physicians from across the country urged us to leave. But though our options had been constrained, they were never nothing. I chose to stay; my faculty all chose to stay. And in the election of November 2023, we fought back.

16 IN CONCLUSION: TREATING THE PAIN OF INDECISION

Doctors likely have over one hundred words for pain. There are the common pseudonyms, then specific words for different organ systems or causes. The suffix *-algia* can be added to essentially any root to make words designating pain in that location: *arthralgia* for pain in one's joints, *neuralgia* for pain originating from neurons, *myalgia* for pain in one's muscles. In addition to location and origin, pain also comes in a range of intensities, frequencies, and flavors: aching, burning, stinging, throbbing. Part of a medical student's acquired competency is fluency in pain's lexicon, necessary for translating critical information between patient and physician. Further complicating matters is the fact that many words have variable if not contradictory meanings. Take, for example, *agony* or *torture*. Both can signal immense, raw, physical pain. But they can also reflect mental states or even just decision paralysis. One may anguish over the choices to be made or be tortured by past alternatives. In addition, *torture* has specific legal definitions in the context of inflicted suffering. Under these definitions, does forced pregnancy continuation formally constitute torture?

This exact question has been given legal consideration by the United Nations' Committee Against Torture (CAT) and the Human Rights Committee (HRC). In 2001, Karen Llantoy was seventeen years old and living in Lima, Peru, when an obstetric ultrasound diagnosed the absence of a fully developed fetal brain. Peru's strict abortion ban held no exceptions for fetal conditions, including those that were lethal. Her physicians nevertheless requested an exception from the health minister due to both Karen Llantoy being under eighteen and the severity of the condition. A psychiatrist, Dr. Marta B. Rondón, submitted a report citing the psychological risks of compelling a minor to continue with a lethal fetal prognosis. The court denied the request, and Karen Llantoy was forced into the third trimester and then delivery, after which, predictably, her child died and she entered a deep state of depression. The HRC later investigated Karen Llantoy's case and found that the Peruvian government had violated her rights of protection against torture and cruelty.[1] They issued financial reparations for her suffering, which were later paid. Similar legal cases asserting torture and cruelty have also been successful in Poland and Ireland.

At this moment, cases identical to that of Karen Llantoy are occurring in the United States, with many abortion bans not holding exceptions for either minors or life-limiting fetal conditions. So are our physicians and legislators right now legally abetting widespread torture?

Torture lacks a single universal definition, with criteria varying from country to country and among different organizations. In the US, the Department of Justice defines torture as "acts specifically intended to inflict severe physical or mental pain or suffering," though this definition is explicitly limited to events outside the United States itself.[2] Amnesty International defines torture as happening "when somebody in an official capacity inflicts severe mental or physical pain or suffering on somebody else for a specific purpose."[3] Despite disparate elements, common criteria for torture entail pain of tremendous severity, be it either mental or physical, the infliction of which is the intentional action of someone in a position of power. By these definitions, how could forced pregnancy continuation not constitute torture?

In states currently enforcing bans without exceptions then, how many individuals are now engaged in torture? The governors and the legislators? The attorney generals? The judges ruling against patients? But what about the doctors, the actual individuals not providing care? The law may clearly prohibit abortion, but obeying the law is a choice one makes. Furthermore, in legal grey zones, we choose which risks we are willing to assume. And how many of our history books are filled with those who choose against consequences to stand against torture, injustice, and cruelty? The hunger strikes, the objectors sitting in prisons, those willing to sacrifice everything?

This is the unique agony of moral injury; it is what makes the pain of moral injury different than just watching a tragedy unfold over which you have no control, a pedestrian watching cars collide in the street ahead. Moral injury instead overlies our moral choices.

How do physicians respond to moral injury after Dobbs? One response is to allow kindness to yourself and the choices you made, to not weigh yourself more harshly than you would another making the same choice. But an alternative also beckons: to tell yourself you did not, in fact, really have a choice. That you had to obey the law. That the legal jeopardy would have ravaged your livelihood, your family, your colleagues. What of all your other patients for whom you would then be unable to provide care? From a standpoint of consequences, the total negative impact would outweigh the fewer tortured patients continuing against their will. All of this may be true, the decisions made eminently rational given the new world into which we are thrown, but rational choices are still choices. As tempting as this conceptualization may be, this is not the historical moment in which we can pretend we are not making choices.

Like the word *torture*, *agony* can describe intense physical discomfort, such as when one is in agony after breaking a leg in a fall. But the word can also be defined as indecision. A patient in one room may agonize in surgical pain but have a clear vision of their treatment course lying ahead. In another room, a patient may sit quietly, experiencing no physical pain at all, but agonize over their treatment options. For the patient with a broken leg, the doctor may walk in with medication for their pain. In my hand, I may hold a pill—perhaps an anti-inflammatory; in contemporary practice, less often an opioid—but one I can hand to the patient, and they can then swallow it with a glass of water. But what of the second patient? What do I hold in my hand when walking into their room?

Jean-Paul Sartre, in his lecture "Existentialism Is a Humanism," tells the story of a young man, likely a fictional character, who seeks his advice during World War II. As the man's brother had died in the war, he is now his aging mother's sole caretaker. Thus, he is duty-bound to continue living with her, though also hears the call to join the war. Does he remain with his mother, or does he fight the evil threatening his country? The question yields bountiful layers of values, duties, and consequences. Sartre likewise explores the dilemma through multiple angles, though he ultimately concludes that the man can only choose his own answer, telling him: "'You are free, so choose; in other words, invent. No general code of ethics can tell you what you ought to do; there are no signs in this world.'"[4]

The fable is told in pure solemness, the lecture given in 1945 in France at the conclusion of the war itself. But now with the elapse of time, it could also perhaps be more humorously framed. We can imagine a young man agonizing over a choice, then one day remembering that a renowned philosopher lives in the next town over—so why not just ask him what to do? He travels to the city and knocks on Sartre's door, expecting an answer from his years of wisdom and scholarly endeavors. And certainly, if he had knocked on the door of one of history's less modern thinkers, he would have likely received guidance: perhaps an answer rooted in theology, virtue ethics, or even just the internal logic of a categorical imperative. Or even if not a clear answer, he could have received some deontological framework to later guide him to a conclusion. But he instead had the misfortune to knock on Sartre's door and was told that he is free.

In medicine, are our patients sometimes also the young man knocking on Sartre's door? Like the aged philosopher, we have years of expertise, scholarly outputs, and may even have written books. So they drive to our offices seeking guidance; likewise, we explore their cases through multiple angles and inform them of what we know. And certainly, if they had knocked on the door of a paternalistic physician from the past, they would have left with a binary directive. But how often now do we appropriately inform them, as the visit winds to its end, that options exist, and that they are free?

In obstetrics, our most agonizing decisions often center around periviability. *Periviability* is roughly defined as the span of gestational ages between which neonatal outcomes, if the fetus is delivered, range between near certain death and likely survival. Roe originally protected the right of abortion until viability, with governments allowed to regulate after that time, stating in the original decision: "For the stage subsequent to viability the State, in promoting its interest in the potentiality of human life, may, if it chooses, regulate, and even proscribe, abortion except where necessary, in appropriate medical judgment, for the preservation of the life or health of the mother."[5]

As a result, even before Dobbs, legislators sought to numerically quantify viability so as to place a firm ceiling atop rights. Exact numeric depictions, however, are inappropriate for many reasons, including viability being context dependent. For example, at any gestational age, is the fetus normally grown or growth restricted? Is delivery imminent from labor or for an imperiled fetal status? Are there structural or genetic concerns as well as prematurity? Neonatal technology also continues to evolve, and thus periviability is also never static.

In retrospect, why was viability selected as autonomy's limit under Roe? Why should rights start or end before or after a given developmental stage? My opinion and that of many others is that they should not. However, in 1973, at the time of the ruling, this was perhaps of less practical concern as viability was far later than it is now given that pediatric care was less advanced. But the limits of viability continue to move downward with advancing technology. By handcuffing abortion rights to viability, we then see only progressive future diminution.

In crafting statewide ballot initiatives after Dobbs, the question of viability became agonizing. Are amendments advanced that restore Roe's constraints or unlock its metaphorical handcuffs? If the text did not include viability language, would this expose it to attacks during the campaign, then causing it to fail? What then would be the consequences if it failed? But if it passed with viability language, how would this then constrain future care? As amendments are inscribed into state constitutions, they may last for decades as pediatric technology continues to advance. At risk of speculation, what if periviability advances downward for future generations to twenty weeks, then eighteen, then sixteen? Alternatively, what if the amendment fails and instead there are no rights for anyone through those subsequent decades? All trade-offs were terrible, the conversations often uncomfortable, the decision-making agonizing.

The stress of navigating amendments, of course, pales before that of patients confronting periviability itself. What are the choices of a patient about to deliver in the periviable window, perhaps one facing unstoppable preterm labor or for whom the pregnancy has become a threat to maternal life? Such patients decide which treatments they will or will not want after delivery. Neonatal intubation and attachment to a ventilator? IV lines and blood draws? Chest compressions?

If we could project into the future after a periviable birth and know the neonate would not survive despite everything we do, what then would be our course of action? In that scenario, intubation, chest compressions, even the placement of IV lines might all lack purpose as they would not achieve their goal of ensuring survival. In addition, if time is going to be short, then all these interventions would just subtract from the parent and child being together, with the neonate wired to machines and incubators rather than in their parents' arms. Instead, you would focus on comfort and parental bonding; you would not intubate or place IVs or commence with chest compressions.

But in many cases, we know the survival probability is low, but it is also uncertain. Thus, you have to balance interventions and the chance of long-term survival against just peacefully holding the child for the time that you have. It can be an agonizing decision.

Legislators in many states also seek to strip these choices away from us through "born alive" laws. In the months after the Dobbs decision, five statewide votes occurred on subjects of abortion. Of the five, Montana's defeat of LR-131 may have received the least fanfare, being more tangentially related to abortion and instead focused on pediatric care after delivery. The ostensible aim was to address the profoundly uncommon cases in which a fetus is born alive after a *termination induction*—that is, when, rather than a surgical procedure, medications are administered to end the pregnancy by inducing labor. However, the language was written broadly enough to cover all cases of pre- and periviable deliveries, essentially criminalizing palliative and comfort care. The amendment stated: "'Born alive' means the complete expulsion or extraction from the mother of a human infant, at any stage of development, who, after expulsion or extraction, breathes, has a beating heart, or has definite movement of voluntary muscles, regardless of whether the umbilical cord has been cut and regardless of whether the expulsion or extraction occurs as a result of natural or induced labor, cesarean section, induced abortion, or another method."[6]

Opponents specifically noted the words "at any stage of development." Thus, as written, the law would apply to preterm labor at eighteen or twenty weeks, gestational ages at which neonatal survival is currently impossible; the provision of chest compressions, intravenous blood draws, or any life-sustaining measure at that gestation is cruelly farcical.

What actions does the law dictate in such deliveries? "A health care provider who is present at the time a born-alive infant is born shall take all medically appropriate and reasonable actions to preserve the life and health of the infant."[7] As is often the case, failure to do so held criminal penalties against physicians.

Supporters claimed that the amendment's intended focus was abortion and not compassionate palliative or comfort care. However, that is not the way it was written, and legally the language would always just be the language.

Fundamentally, "born alive" laws are another assault to autonomy, the belief that in agonizing situations the legislators will supersede the parents, that they will make these decisions rather than us. Dobbs likewise not only curtails abortion rights but also, as illustrated here and elsewhere, threatens to expand outward, including into our pediatric care after delivery. In 2022, Montana voters rejected the amendment.

Without "born alive" laws, would physicians then not provide care to neonates? No, because physicians always provide care; we just provide care in alignment with our patients' varying goals. If the parents' goals after a periviable delivery are to optimize the prolongation of life, then physicians perform care in alignment with those goals. If, however, the goals of the parents are comfort, then the physicians provide care in alignment with those goals. But in neither situation do we not provide care. These laws thus never enhance care: They just force the goals of care to be those of the legislators over those of the parents.

Say that an older man with a life-threatening disease worsens despite a third treatment attempt. He must now choose his options and choose his goals. If his goal remains a potential cure, or at least the prolongation of life, then treatments aligning with that goal may include complicated surgeries or enrollment in research trials, time spent in hospitals or clinics rather than at home or among friends. Instead, his primary goal may be comfort and optimizing the quality of his remaining time, a goal with which surgeries or experimental treatments may not align. So how does he then make treatment decisions? First, he has to sit and think about his goals. What aspects of the future hold the greatest importance? Even outside of illness or medicine, we all first choose the goals in our lives, then our other options fall in alignment.

In the office, my wife sees a child who, for hypothetical, illustrative purposes, has the same disease, treatment course, prognosis, and options as are faced by the older man. What, then, are the differences in these scenarios? The patient being a child makes the decisions more agonizing, if not tortuous. In the quantification of potential future years, the stakes are numerically far higher, the possibility of cure desperately enticing. Thus, the parents may select goals that differ from the older man's, but in both cases they first agonize over goals and then select treatments in concert with their aims. Do the scenarios thus truly differ in their underlying calculus?

Later in my own office, a patient has a life-limiting fetal anomaly, or in the hospital a periviable patient in preterm labor is about to deliver. These patients must also choose their goals of care, considering, perhaps painfully, which future outcomes they hold highest, contemplating goals of life prolongation and goals of comfort. But does the most fundamental calculus of these decisions also remain the same? And of these three scenarios, why is it this last patient who is now subjugated to legislative interference? Why, after Dobbs, did Montana voters have to cast ballots for or against this patient?

Patients surviving a disease often will later state that they found benefit in their journey in addition to suffering, precisely because they were forced to confront their goals. Perhaps they had wandered through life healthy but inchoate; then suddenly they had to starkly ponder the future they wanted, which aspects of their existence were of importance. Now they know which friends stood with them or wisped away, which of their life's fabrics were sewn with woolen yarn or gossamer thread. But more critically, they now know their aim, the locations in which to place their feet along the trail ahead.

When a patient agonizes in physical pain, I can give them a pill to dissipate discomfort. What if I also held a pill for those agonizing in indecision? Would I hand it to them? Should they swallow it with a glass of water? It is when we agonize that we also contemplate our goals, the future. Medicine, and perhaps the entire country, has agonized after the Dobbs decision. Ideally, it would all stop; ideally, the judicial rulings and bans would all magically disappear after casting some spell. But like someone confronting a medical endangerment, are we also now forced to consider our goals? We cannot build solutions in the present without also knowing the future we want. As a country, what now is our desired future? What are the freedoms that are of greatest collective importance? Right now, I do not know what our direction will be—but we all have to decide.

Acknowledgments

First, I am indebted to my family and kids. I wrote in early mornings and late evenings, on weekends and during hockey practices. Thanks for understanding when I slipped away to libraries and coffee shops, as well as reading drafts and then telling me which portions were terrible. Nothing would also be possible without my wife, who, when reviewing the first drafts, felt odd actually seeing names in print, so everyone was thereafter changed to "wife," "son," or "daughter" rather than actual names. Then I decided, for consistency, to use no real names, except in unavoidable references to public figures. Thus, everyone became a "fellow," a "colleague," a "resident," and so on. So for everyone who knows they were there, everyone who, when reading, also saw themselves in the clinics or operating rooms or legislative halls, thanks for being part of this story. Particular appreciation goes to my colleagues at both the University of Pittsburgh and the University of Rochester, who helped guide us through our difficult pregnancies. I also would never have navigated the storm that followed Dobbs without Kate Connor at the American College of Obstetricians and Gynecologists and the team at the Society for Maternal-Fetal Medicine: Kerri Wade, Rebecca Abbott, and Samantha Berg.

This book's genesis was an essay I wrote for *The New York Times* shortly after the Dobbs decision, for which I am grateful to opinion editor Lauren Kelley. After publication of that essay, I was contacted by my now agent, Jennifer Weis. I had never previously considered writing a book, so I am forever appreciative of her both having the vision to see this story and guiding me through a process about which I originally knew nothing. Throughout this course, editor Shannon O'Neill has provided critical insights and guidance, as well as a fundamental belief in the project.

When I first considered writing, one of my first calls was to fellow MFM specialist Dr. Chavi Karkowsky, author of the book *High Risk*, which is recommended for anyone wanting to further learn about our subspeciality. She gave me a crash course in, well, writing and publishing. Before submitting my first complete draft, I nervously sent it to two trusted colleagues: Dr. Cara Heuser and Dr. Amy Burkett. As busy clinicians, it is a tall ask to read an entire book in a short time frame and then provide crucial insights.

My appreciation goes to everyone at the MIT Press, particularly Bob Prior, Janice Audet, and my anonymous reviewers. Bob supported this book even through a significant heath event. He later retired after a long career, making this one of his last acquisitions. I hope he is enjoying reading it somewhere. Janice then picked up the reins, resulting in significant improvements from a fresh set of eyes.

Ohio's reproductive freedom amendment, passed by voters in 2023, hung over much of this writing. Importantly, this is not intended as the story of the voter amendment itself, as that is not my own story to tell; it belongs instead to the legions who labored to bring it to the ballot and succeed: the volunteers collecting signatures, the campaign strategists, the lawyers who fought diligently in the courtrooms, and the leaders of Ohio Physicians for Reproductive Rights and Ohioans for Reproductive Freedom (now Abortion Forward).

Finally, appreciation goes to my colleagues in Cleveland and Ohio and perhaps the entire field of obstetrics and gynecology. It is difficult to imagine any medical specialty enduring a one-two punch equivalent to the COVID pandemic followed immediately by Dobbs. But through both, we hung together in Cleveland, in Ohio, and across the country. In neither case did we choose these fights, but you never choose your history—only how you choose to respond.

Notes

CHAPTER 1

1. Nichole Nidey, Sina Haeri, and Andrea L. Greiner, "Examining Geographic Access to Maternal-Fetal Medicine Care Across the United States," *American Journal of Obstetrics & Gynecology* 226, no. 1 (2002): S564, https://doi.org/10.1016/j.ajog.2021.11.934.

2. Scott A. Sullivan, Elizabeth G. Hill, Roger B. Newman, and M. Kathryn Menard, "Maternal-Fetal Medicine Specialist Density Is Inversely Associated with Maternal Mortality Ratios," *American Journal of Obstetrics & Gynecology* 193, no. 3 (2005): 1083–1108, https://doi.org/10.1016/j.ajog.2005.05.085.

3. American Academy of Pediatrics and American College of Obstetricians and Gynecologists, *Guidelines for Perinatal Care*, 8th ed. (ACOG Publications, 2017), https://doi.org/10.1542/9781610020886.

4. Sarahn M. Wheeler, Sabrena O. Myers, Geeta K. Swamy, and Evan R. Myers, "Estimated Prevalence of Risk Factors for Preeclampsia Among Individuals Giving Birth in the US in 2019," *JAMA Network Open* 5, no. 1 (2022): e2142343, https://doi.org/10.1001/jamanetworkopen.2021.42343.

5. Valery A. Danilack, Anthony P. Nunes, and Maureen G. Phipps, "Unexpected Complications of Low-Risk Pregnancies in the United States," *American Journal of Obstetrics & Gynecology* 212, no. 6 (2015): 809.e1–6, https://doi.org/10.1016/j.ajog.2015.03.038.

CHAPTER 2

1. See https://www.legislature.ohio.gov/legislation/133/sb23.

2. See https://ldh.la.gov/assets/oph/Rulemaking/er/LDH_ER_List_of_Conditions_that_Shall_Deem_an_Unborn_Child_Medically_Futile_CLV_Signed_and_Dated_1_August_2022.pdf.

3. Alison Marie Bauer, Justin Lappen, and David Hackney, "Pregnancy Outcomes in Peri-Menarchal Adolescents," *Obstetrics & Gynecology* 133 (2019): 64S, https://doi.org/10.1097/01.AOG.0000559040.56251.c9.

4. Abigail Adcox, "Ohio AG Hasn't Heard 'Whisper' of Evidence for Child Rape Victim Seeking Abortion," *Washington Examiner*, July 12, 2022, https://www.washingtonexaminer.com/news/227109/ohio-ag-hasnt-heard-whisper-of-evidence-for-child-rape-victim-seeking-abortion.

CHAPTER 3

1. Kavitha Surana, "Abortion Bans Have Delayed Emergency Medical Care. In Georgia, Experts Say This Mother's Death Was Preventable," ProPublica, September 16, 2024, https://www.propublica.org/article/georgia-abortion-ban-amber-thurman-death.

CHAPTER 4

1. Jeremy Pelzer, "Ohio Lawmaker Not Giving Up Longshot Quest to Arrest Gov. Mike DeWine over Coronavirus Orders," *Cleveland Plain Dealer*, October 7, 2020, https://www.cleveland.com/open/2020/10/ohio-lawmaker-not-giving-up-longshot-quest-to-arrest-gov-mike-dewine-over-coronavirus-orders.html.
2. See https://www.legislature.ohio.gov/legislation/133/hb413.
3. Jessica Glenza, "Ohio Bill Orders Doctors to 'Reimplant Ectopic Pregnancy' or Face 'Abortion Murder' Charges," *The Guardian*, November 29, 2019, https://www.theguardian.com/us-news/2019/nov/29/ohio-extreme-abortion-bill-reimplant-ectopic-pregnancy.
4. Andrew J. Tobias, "Secretary of State Frank LaRose Says Abortion Opponents Helped Craft Ballot Language to Aid Defeat of Issue 1," *Cleveland Plain Dealer*, November 29, 2023, https://www.cleveland.com/news/2023/11/secretary-of-state-frank-larose-says-abortion-opponents-helped-craft-ballot-language-to-aid-defeat-of-issue-1.html.
5. "Letter Opposing November Amendment," Archdiocese of Cincinnati, August 12, 2023, https://catholicaoc.org/news/press-releases/letter-opposing-november-amendment.
6. Kate Zernike and Lisa Lerer, "Why the Abortion Ballot Question in Ohio Is Confusing Voters," *New York Times*, November 2, 2023, https://www.nytimes.com/2023/11/02/us/abortion-ballot-ohio-vote.html.

CHAPTER 5

1. Shilpa Jindia, "Belly of the Beast: California's Dark History of Forced Sterilizations," *The Guardian*, June 30, 2020, https://www.theguardian.com/us-news/2020/jun/30/california-prisons-forced-sterilizations-belly-beast.
2. See https://www.casemine.com/judgement/us/59148e7dadd7b04934554f28.
3. See https://law.justia.com/cases/illinois/court-of-appeals-first-appellate-district/1997/1962316.html.
4. See https://law.justia.com/cases/illinois/court-of-appeals-first-appellate-district/1997/1962316.html.

5. See https://law.justia.com/cases/illinois/court-of-appeals-first-appellate-district/1997/1962316.html.

6. Marcela Valdes, "When Doctors Took 'Family Planning' into Their Own Hands," *New York Times*, February 1, 2016, https://www.nytimes.com/2016/02/01/magazine/when-doctors-took-family-planning-into-their-own-hands.html.

7. Andrew J. Tobias, "Secretary of State Frank LaRose Says Abortion Opponents Helped Craft Ballot Language to Aid Defeat of Issue 1," *Cleveland Plain Dealer*, updated January 30, 2024, https://www.cleveland.com/news/2023/11/secretary-of-state-frank-larose-says-abortion-opponents-helped-craft-ballot-language-to-aid-defeat-of-issue-1.html.

8. See https://www.supremecourt.ohio.gov/pdf_viewer/pdf_viewer.aspx?pdf=948819.pdf&subdirectory=2023-1088%5CDocketItems&source=DL_Clerk.

9. See https://www.ohiosos.gov/globalassets/ballotboard/2023/certified-language-9-21-ballot-board.pdf.

10. See https://www.supremecourt.ohio.gov/pdf_viewer/pdf_viewer.aspx?pdf=949015.pdf&subdirectory=2023-1088%5CDocketItems&source=DL_Clerk.

11. See https://www.supremecourt.ohio.gov/pdf_viewer/pdf_viewer.aspx?pdf=949015.pdf&subdirectory=2023-1088%5CDocketItems&source=DL_Clerk.

12. Kate Kelly and David Perlmutt, "Inside the Party Switch That Blew Up North Carolina Politics," *New York Times*, July 30, 2023, https://www.nytimes.com/2023/07/30/us/inside-the-party-switch-that-blew-up-north-carolina-politics.html.

CHAPTER 6

1. Sarah McCammon and Lauren Hodges, "Doctors' Worst Fears About the Texas Abortion Law Are Coming True," *All Things Considered*, NPR, March 1, 2022.

2. Susan Tebben, "Another Abortion Ban Hits Ohio House, Depends on Roe v. Wade," *Ohio Capital Journal*, March 17, 2022, https://ohiocapitaljournal.com/2022/03/17/another-abortion-ban-hits-ohio-house-depends-on-roe-v-wade/.

3. Anjali Nambiar, Shivani Patel, Patricia Santiago-Munoz, Catherine Y. Spong, and David B. Nelson, "Maternal Morbidity and Fetal Outcomes Among Pregnant Women at 22 Weeks' Gestation or Less with Complications in 2 Texas Hospitals After Legislation on Abortion," *American Journal of Obstetrics & Gynecology* 227, no. 4 (2022): 648–650.el, https://doi.org/10.1016/j.ajog.2022.06.060.

CHAPTER 7

1. "ACOG Committee Opinion No. 762: Prepregnancy Counseling," *Obstetrics & Gynecology* 133, no. 1 (2019): e78–e89, https://doi.org/10.1097/AOG.0000000000003013.

2. See https://www.ansirh.org/research/ongoing/turnaway-study.

3. Clifton Fadiman, *Enter, Conversing* (Cleveland, OH: The World Publishing Company, 1962), 109.

4. Mary Catherine Beach, Somnath Saha, Jenny Park, Janiece Taylor, Paul Drew, Eve Plank, et al., "Testimonial Injustice: Linguistic Bias in the Medical Records of Black Patients and Women," *Journal of General Internal Medicine* 36 (2021): 1708–1714, https://doi.org/10.1007/s11606-021-06682-z.

CHAPTER 8

1. "Committee Opinion No. 614: Management of Pregnant Women with Presumptive Exposure to Listeria Monocytogenes," *Obstetrics & Gynecology* 124, no. 6 (2014): 1241–1244, https://doi.org/10.1097/01.AOG.0000457501.73326.6c.

2. Benjamin Haynes, Debra Houry, Laura Bachmann, Stephanie Taylor, and the Centers for Disease Control and Prevention, "Transcript for Vital Signs Telebriefing: Syphilis in Babies Reflects Health System Failures," *CDC Vital Signs*, November 7, 2023, https://stacks.cdc.gov/view/cdc/135317.

3. American College of Obstetricians and Gynecologists, *Screening in Syphilis in Pregnancy 2024*, Practice Advisory, April 2024, https://www.acog.org/clinical/clinical-guidance/practice-advisory/articles/2024/04/screening-for-syphilis-in-pregnancy.

4. "Practice Bulletin No. 151: Cytomegalovirus, Parvovirus B19, Varicella Zoster, and Toxoplasmosis in Pregnancy," *Obstetrics & Gynecology* 125, no. 6 (June 2015): 1510–1525, https://doi.org/10.1097/01.AOG.0000466430.19823.53.

5. Giovanni Nigro, Stuart P. Adler, Renato La Torre, and Al M. Best, for the Congenital Cytomegalovirus Collaborating Group, "Passive Immunization During Pregnancy for Congenital Cytomegalovirus Infection," *New England Journal of Medicine* 353, no. 13 (2005): 1350–1362, https://doi.org/10.1056/NEJMoa043337.

6. Brenna L. Hughes, Rebecca G. Clifton, Dwight J. Rouse, George R. Saade, Mara J. Dinsmoor, Uma M. Reddy, et al., "A Trial of Hyperimmune Globulin to Prevent Congenital Cytomegalovirus Infection," *New England Journal of Medicine* 385, no. 5 (2021): 436–444, https://doi.org/10.1056/NEJMoa1913569.

7. Keren Shahar-Nissan, Joseph Pardo, Orit Peled, Irit Krause, Efraim Bilavsky, Arnon Wiznitzer, et al., "Valaciclovir to Prevent Vertical Transmission of Cytomegalovirus After Maternal Primary Infection During Pregnancy: A Randomised, Double-Blind, Placebo-Controlled Trial," *The Lancet* 396, no. 10253 (2020): 779–785, https://doi.org/10.1016/S0140-6736(20)31868-7.

8. See https://www.nationalcmv.org.

CHAPTER 9

1. Lizzie Presser and Kavitha Surana, "A Third Woman Died Under Texas' Abortion Ban. Doctors Are Avoiding D&Cs and Reaching for Riskier Miscarriage Treatments," ProPublica,

November 25, 2024, https://www.propublica.org/article/porsha-ngumezi-miscarriage-death-texas-abortion-ban.

2. David N. Hackney and J. Christopher Glantz, "Vaginal Bleeding in Early Pregnancy and Preterm Birth: Systemic Review and Analysis of Heterogeneity," *Journal of Maternal-Fetal & Neonatal Medicine* 24, no. 6 (2011): 778–786, https://doi.org/10.3109/14767058.2010.530707.

3. Israel Thaler, Dorit Manor, Joseph Itskovitz, Shraga Rottem, Nathan Levit, Ilan Timor-Tritsch, et al., "Changes in Uterine Blood Flow During Human Pregnancy," *American Journal of Obstetrics & Gynecology* 162, no. 1 (1990): 121–125, https://doi.org/10.1016/0002-9378(90)90834-T.

CHAPTER 10

1. Erin B. Stallings, Jennifer L. Isenburg, Rachel E. Rutkowski, Russell S. Kirby, Wendy N. Nembhard, Theresa Sandidge, et al., "National Population-Based Estimates for Major Birth Defects, 2016–2020," *Birth Defects Research* 116, no. 1 (2024): e2301, https://doi.org/10.1002/bdr2.2301.

2. Francis Stead Sellers, "Her Baby Has a Deadly Diagnosis. Her Florida Doctors Refused an Abortion," *Washington Post*, May 19, 2023, https://www.washingtonpost.com/health/2023/02/18/florida-abortion-ban-unviable-pregnancy-potter-syndrome/.

3. Elizabeth Cohen, Carma Hassan, and Amanda Musa, "Because of Florida Abortion Laws, She Carried Her Baby to Term Knowing He Would Die," CNN Health, May 3, 2023, https://www.cnn.com/2023/05/02/health/florida-abortion-term-pregnancy.

4. Marieke F. J. Buijtendijk, Bo B. Bet, Mariska M. G. Leeflang, Harsha Shah, Tom Reuvekamp, Timothy Goring, et al., "Diagnostic Accuracy of Ultrasound Screening for Fetal Structural Abnormalities During the First and Second Trimester of Pregnancy in Low-Risk and Unselected Populations," *Cochrane Database of Systematic Reviews*, no. 5 (2024): CD014715, https://doi.org/10.1002/14651858.CD014715.pub2.

5. Neelam Bohra, "'They're Just Going to Let Me Die?' One Woman's Abortion Odyssey," *New York Times*, August 1, 2022, https://www.nytimes.com/2022/08/01/us/abortion-journey-crossing-states.html.

CHAPTER 11

1. Jasmine D. Johnson and Judette M. Louis, "Does Race or Ethnicity Play a Role in the Origin, Pathophysiology, and Outcomes of Preeclampsia? An Expert Review of the Literature," *American Journal of Obstetrics & Gynecology* 226, no. 2S (2022): S876–S885, https://doi.org/10.1016/j.ajog.2020.07.038.

2. Sara Hammel, "Mariah Carey: I Lost 70 Lbs. After Twins," *People*, November 2011.

3. Clover Hope, "Beyoncé in Her Own Words: Her Life, Her Body, Her Heritage," *Vogue*, September 2018.

4. Margaret Osborne, "What Is Eclampsia? Olympian Tori Bowie May Have Died from the Rare Pregnancy Condition," *Smithsonian Magazine*, June 16, 2023, https://www.smithsonianmag.com/smart-news/what-is-eclampsia-olympian-tori-bowie-may-have-died-from-the-rare-pregnancy-condition-180982388/.

5. See https://web.archive.org/web/20191201090254/https://www.cdc.gov/reproductivehealth/maternal-mortality/pregnancy-mortality-surveillance-system.htm.

6. Michelle Rodrigues, "The Absurd Pregnancy Math Behind the 'Six-Week' Abortion Ban," *Scientific American*, September 4, 2021, https://www.scientificamerican.com/article/the-absurd-pregnancy-math-behind-the-lsquo-six-week-rsquo-abortion-ban/.

CHAPTER 12

1. Cary Funk, Meg Hefferon, Brian Kennedy, and Courtney Johnson, "4. Americans Generally View Medical Professionals Favorably, but About Half Consider Misconduct a Big Problem," in *Trust and Mistrust in Americans' Views of Scientific Experts* (Pew Research Center, August 2, 2019), https://www.pewresearch.org/science/2019/08/02/americans-generally-view-medical-professionals-favorably-but-about-half-consider-misconduct-a-big-problem/.

2. Anjali Nambiar, Shivani Patel, Patricia Santiago-Munoz, Catherine Y. Spong, and David B. Nelson, "Maternal Morbidity and Fetal Outcomes Among Pregnant Women at 22 Weeks' Gestation or Less with Complications in 2 Texas Hospitals After Legislation on Abortion," *American Journal of Obstetrics & Gynecology* 227, no. 4 (2022): 648–650.el, https://doi.org/10.1016/j.ajog.2022.06.060.

3. Elizabeth Cohen, Justin Lape, and Danielle Herman, "'Heartbreaking' Stories Go Untold, Doctors Say, as Employers 'Muzzle' Them in Wake of Abortion Ruling," CNN Health, October 12, 2022, https://www.cnn.com/2022/10/12/health/abortion-doctors-talking.

CHAPTER 13

1. Gregory Krieg, "'Don't Piss Women Off': Democrat John Fetterman Makes Abortion Rights Push in Philadelphia Suburbs," CNN Politics, September 11, 2022, https://www.cnn.com/2022/09/11/politics/john-fetterman-mehmet-oz-pennsylvania-senate-race-abortion.

2. Ava Sasani and Sheryl Gay Stolberg, "Indiana Attorney General Asks Medical Board to Discipline Abortion Doctor," *New York Times*, November 30, 2022, https://www.nytimes.com/2022/11/30/us/indiana-attorney-general-abortion-doctor.html.

3. Tom McGrath, *Megamind* (DreamWorks Animation, 2010).

4. Jane Spencer and Christina Jewett, "12 Months of Trauma: More Than 3,600 US Health Workers Died in Covid's First Year," KFF Health News, April 8, 2021, https://kffhealthnews.org/news/article/us-health-workers-deaths-covid-lost-on-the-frontline/.

5. See "ICN Says 115,000 Healthcare Worker Deaths from COVID-19 Exposes Collective Failure of Leaders to Protect Global Workforce," ICN, October 21, 2021, https://www.icn.ch/news/icn-says-115000-healthcare-worker-deaths-covid-19-exposes-collective-failure-leaders-protect.
6. Mathew V. Kiang, Lindsey E. Carlasare, Sonoo Thadaney Israni, John J. Norcini, Junaid A. B. Zaman, and Kirsten Bibbins-Domingo, "Excess Mortality Among US Physicians During the COVID-19 Pandemic," *JAMA Internal Medicine* 183, no. 4 (2023): 374–376, https://doi.org/10.1001/jamainternmed.2022.6308.
7. Leonard J. Hoenig, "In Memoriam: Physicians Who Have Died of COVID-19 in the United States," *Clinics in Dermatology* 38, no. 6 (2020): 771–772, https://doi.org/10.1016/j.clindermatol.2020.05.017.
8. Steven J. Scheinman, Patrick Fleming, and Kellyann Niotis, "Oath Taking at U.S. and Canadian Medical School Ceremonies: Historical Perspectives, Current Practices, and Future Considerations," *Academic Medicine* 93, no. 9 (2018): 1301–1306, https://doi.org/10.1097/ACM.0000000000002097.
9. Louis Lasagna, "Would Hippocrates Rewrite His Oath?," *New York Times*, June 28, 1964, https://www.nytimes.com/1964/06/28/archives/would-hippocrates-rewrite-his-oath-after-2000-years-the-greek.html.
10. See https://www.supremecourt.gov/pdfs/transcripts/1972/70-18_10-11-1972.pdf.
11. Benjamin Watson, "It's Time to Stop Playing Word Games. Abortion Isn't Health Care | Opinion," *Newsweek*, March 11, 2022, https://www.newsweek.com/its-time-stop-playing-word-games-abortion-isnt-health-care-opinion-1686044.
12. Mary Kekatos, "Why Doctors Say the 'Save the Mother's Life' Exception of Abortion Bans Is Medically Risky," ABC News, June 13, 2022, https://abcnews.go.com/Health/doctors-save-mothers-life-exception-abortion-bans-medically/story?id=84668658.
13. See the AMA Code of Medical Ethics at https://code-medical-ethics.ama-assn.org/preface-preamble.
14. Matthew K. Wynia, "Professional Civil Disobedience—Medical-Society Responsibilities After *Dobbs*," *New England Journal of Medicine* 387, no. 11 (2022): 959–961, https://doi.org/10.1056/NEJMp2210192.

CHAPTER 14

1. See https://www.txcourts.gov/media/1457645/230994pc.pdf.
2. See https://www.txcourts.gov/media/1457645/230994pc.pdf.
3. See https://www.txcourts.gov/media/1457645/230994pc.pdf.
4. J. David Goodman, "Abortion Ruling Keeps Texas Doctors Afraid of Prosecution," *New York Times*, December 13, 2023, https://www.nytimes.com/2023/12/13/us/texas-abortion-doctor-prosecution.html.

5. See https://texhealthlaw.org/texas-register-april-5-2024-volume-49-number-14/#:~:text=New%20§165.9%2C%20titled%20Complaints,independent%20of%20any%20Board%20decision.

6. See https://www150.statcan.gc.ca/n1/daily-quotidien/240925/dq240925c-eng.htm.

CHAPTER 15

1. Angela Palermo, "Idaho Has Lost 22% of Its Practicing Obstetricians in the Last 15 Months, Report Says," *Idaho Statesman*, May 15, 2024, https://www.idahostatesman.com/living/health-fitness/article285692341.html.

2. Ashley Stoneburner, Ripley Lucas, Jazmin Fontenot, Christina Brigance, Erin Jones, and Andrea L. DeMaria, *Nowhere to Go: Maternity Care Deserts Across the US*, Report No 4 (March of Dimes, 2024), https://www.marchofdimes.org/maternity-care-deserts-report.

CHAPTER 16

1. See https://digitallibrary.un.org/record/575355?ln=en&v=pdf.

2. See "20. Torture (18 U.S.C. 2340A)," in *Criminal Resource Manual* (US Department of Justice, accessed October 30, 2025), https://www.justice.gov/archives/jm/criminal-resource-manual-20-torture-18-usc-2340a#:~:text=Torture%20is%20defined%20to%20include,suffering%20incidental%20to%20lawful%20sanctions.

3. See "Torture," Amnesty International, accessed October 30, 2025, https://www.amnesty.org/en/what-we-do/torture/#:~:text=Torture%20is%20when%20somebody%20in,to%20get%20information%20from%20them.

4. Jean-Paul Sartre, *Existentialism Is a Humanism*, trans. Carol Macomber (New Haven: Yale University Press, 2007), 33.

5. See https://tile.loc.gov/storage-services/service/ll/usrep/usrep410/usrep410113/usrep410113.pdf.

6. See https://archive.legmt.gov/bills/2021/billhtml/HB0167.htm.

7. See https://archive.legmt.gov/bills/2021/billhtml/HB0167.htm.

Suggested Reading

CHAPTER 1

D'Alton, Mary, Star Poole, and Rebecca Rinehard. *Society of Perinatal Obstetricians: The First Two Decades*. Society of Perinatal Obstetricians, 1997.

Karkowsky, Chavi Eve. *High Risk: A Doctor's Notes on Pregnancy, Birth and the Unexpected*. Liverlight, 2020.

Lo, W. Y., and J. M. Friedman. "Teratogenicity of Recently Introduced Medications in Human Pregnancy." *Obstetrics & Gynecology* 100, no. 3 (2002):465–467.

Lowe, Jamie. "What a High-Risk Pregnancy Looks Like After Dobbs." *New York Times*, September 13, 2022.

CHAPTER 2

Eaton, Sabrina. "Arrest Prompts Criticism of Republicans Like AG Dave Yost Who Questioned Story of 10-Year-Old Rape Victim Who Left Ohio to Get an Abortion." *Cleveland Plain Dealer*, July 13, 2022.

Sedgh, Gilda, Lawrence B. Finer, Akinrinola Bankole, Michelle A. Eilers, and Susheela Singh. "Adolescent Pregnancy, Birth, and Abortion Rates Across Countries: Levels and Recent Trends." *Journal of Adolescent Health* 56, no. 2 (Feb 2015): 223–230. https://doi.org/10.1016/j.jadohealth.2014.09.007.

Sleven, Peter. "One of the Last Abortion Doctors in Indiana." *New Yorker*, February 25, 2024.

CHAPTER 3

"Practice Bulletin No. 174: Evaluation and Management of Adnexal Masses." *Obstetrics & Gynecology* 128, no. 5 (November 2016): e210–e226. https://doi.org/10.1097/AOG.0000000000001768.

Schmeler, Kathleen M., William W. Mayo-Smith, Jeffrey F. Peipert, Sherry Weitzen, Misty D. Manuel, and Mary E. Gordinier. Adnexal Masses in Pregnancy: Surgery Compared with Observation. *Obstetrics & Gynecology* 105 (May 2005): 1098–1103. https://doi.org/10.1097/01.AOG.0000157465.99639.e5.

Surana, Kavitha. "Abortion Bans Have Delayed Emergency Medical Care. In Georgia, Experts Say This Mother's Death Was Preventable." ProPublica, September 16, 2024. https://www.propublica.org/article/georgia-abortion-ban-amber-thurman-death.

CHAPTER 4

Glenza, Jessica. "Ohio Bill Orders Doctors to 'Reimplant Ectopic Pregnancy' or Face 'Abortion Murder' Charges." *The Guardian*, November 29, 2019.

Karlis, Nicole. "'Reckless' and 'Unsafe': The Misinformation Around 'Late-Term Abortion' Is Harmful, Experts Say." *Salon*, July 12, 2024. https://www.salon.com/2024/07/12/reckless-and-unsafe-the-misinformation-around-late-term-abortion-is-harmful-experts-say/.

"Viral Hepatitis in Pregnancy: ACOG Clinical Practice Guideline No. 6." *Obstetrics & Gynecology* 142, no. 3 (September 2023): 745–759. https://doi.org/10.1097/AOG.0000000000005300.

CHAPTER 5

Hackney, David. "Abortion Rights Have Been Winning. Ohio Leaders Are Trying to Change That." *New York Times*, November 5, 2023.

Hallman, J. C. *Say Anarcha: A Young Woman, a Devious Surgeon, and the Harrowing Birth of Modern Women's Health*. Henry Holt and Company, 2023.

Kelly, Kate and Perlmutt. "Inside the Party Switch That Blew Up North Carolina Politics" *New York Times*, July 2023.

CHAPTER 6

Nambiar, Anjali, Shivani Patel, Patricia Santiago-Munoz, Catherine Y. Spong, and David B. Nelson. "Maternal Morbidity and Fetal Outcomes Among Pregnant Women at 22 Weeks' Gestation or Less with Complications in 2 Texas Hospitals After Legislation on Abortion." *American Journal of Obstetrics & Gynecology* 227, no. 4 (October 2022): 648–650el. https://doi.org/10.1016/j.ajog.2022.06.060.

"Prelabor Rupture of Membranes: ACOG Practice Bulletin, Number 217." *Obstetrics & Gynecology* 135, no. 3 (March 2020): e80–e97. https://doi.org/10.1097/AOG.0000000000003700.

Winn, Hung N., Michael Chen, Erol Amon, Terry L. Leet, Joseph B. Shumway, and Dorothea Mostello. "Neonatal Pulmonary Hypoplasia and Perinatal Mortality in Patients with Midtrimester Rupture of Amniotic Membranes—a Critical Analysis." *American Journal of Obstetrics & Gynecology* 182, no. 6 (June 2000): 1638–1644.

CHAPTER 7

Beach, Mary Catherine, Somnath Saha, Jenny Park, Janiece Taylor, Paul Drew, Eve Plank, Lisa A. Cooper, and Brant Chee. "Testimonial Injustice: Linguistic Bias in the Medical Records of Black

Patients and Women." *Journal of General Internal Medicine* 36 (2021): 1708–1714. https://doi.org/10.1007/s11606-021-06682-z.

Compston, Alastair, and Alasdair Coles. "Multiple Sclerosis." *Lancet* 372, no. 9648 (2008): 1502–1517. https://doi.org/10.1016/S0140-6736(08)61620-7.

Foster, Diana Greene. *The Turnaway Study: Ten Years, a Thousand Women, and the Consequences of Having—or Being Denied—an Abortion*. Scribner, 2020.

Krysko, Kristen M., Ruth Dobson, Raed Alroughani, Maria Pia Amato, Riley Bove, Andrea I. Ciplea, et al. "Family Planning Considerations in People with Multiple Sclerosis." *Lancet Neurology* 22, no. 4 (April 2023): 350–366. https://doi.org/10.1016/S1474-4422(22)00426-4.

Salani, Ritu, Caroline C. Billingsley, and Sarah M. Crafton. "Cancer and Pregnancy: An Overview for Obstetricians and Gynecologists." *American Journal of Obstetrics & Gynecology* 211, no. 1 (July 2014): 7–14.

CHAPTER 8

Hughes, Brenna L., Rebecca G. Clifton, Dwight J. Rouse, George R. Saade, Mara J. Dinsmoor, Uma M. Reddy, et al. "A Trial of Hyperimmune Globulin to Prevent Congenital Cytomegalovirus Infection." *New England Journal of Medicine* 385, no. 5 (2021): 436–444. https://doi.org/10.1056/NEJMoa1913569.

Nigro, Giovanni, Stuart P. Adler, Renato La Torre, and Al M. Best, for the Congenital Cytomegalovirus Collaborating Group. "Passive Immunization During Pregnancy for Congenital Cytomegalovirus Infection." *New England Journal of Medicine* 353, no. 13 (2005): 1350–1362. https://doi.org/10.1056/NEJMoa043337.

Shahar-Nissan, Keren, Joseph Pardo, Orit Peled, Irit Krause, Efraim Bilavsky, Arnon Wiznitzer, et al. "Valaciclovir to Prevent Vertical Transmission of Cytomegalovirus After Maternal Primary Infection During Pregnancy: A Randomised, Double-Blind, Placebo-Controlled Trial." *Lancet* 396, no. 10253 (2020): 779–785. https://doi.org/10.1016/S0140-6736(20)31868-7.

CHAPTER 9

Hackney, David N., and J. Christopher Glantz. "Vaginal Bleeding in Early Pregnancy and Preterm Birth: Systemic Review and Analysis of Heterogeneity." *Journal of Maternal-Fetal & Neonatal Medicine* 24, no. 6 (2011): 778–786. https://doi.org/10.3109/14767058.2010.530707.

Mendez-Figueroa, Hector, Joshua D. Dahlke, Roxanne A. Vrees, and Dwight J. Rouse. "Trauma in Pregnancy: An Updated Systematic Review." *American Journal of Obstetrics & Gynecology* 209, no. 1 (July 2013): 1–10. https://doi.org/10.1016/j.ajog.2013.01.021.

Presser, Lizzie, and Kavitha Surana. "A Third Woman Died Under Texas' Abortion Ban. Doctors Are Avoiding D&Cs and Reaching for Riskier Miscarriage Treatments." ProPublica, November 25, 2024. https://www.propublica.org/article/porsha-ngumezi-miscarriage-death-texas-abortion-ban.

CHAPTER 10

Buijtendijk, Marieke F. J., Bo B. Bet, Mariska M. G. Leeflang, Harsha Shah, Tom Reuvekamp, Timothy Goring, et al. "Diagnostic Accuracy of Ultrasound Screening for Fetal Structural Abnormalities During the First and Second Trimester of Pregnancy in Low-Risk and Unselected Populations." *Cochrane Database of Systematic Reviews*, no. 5 (2024): Article CD014715. https://doi.org/10.1002/14651858.CD014715.pub2.

Sellers, Frances Stead. "Her Baby Has a Deadly Diagnosis. Her Florida Doctors Refused an Abortion." *Washington Post*, May 19, 2023. https://www.washingtonpost.com/health/2023/02/18/florida-abortion-ban-unviable-pregnancy-potter-syndrome/.

Yang, Maya. "Texas Women Give Harrowing Testimony on Impact of Extreme Abortion Ban." *The Guardian*, July 20, 2023. https://www.theguardian.com/us-news/2023/jul/20/texas-women-pregnancy-abortion-ban.

CHAPTER 11

"Gestational Hypertension and Preeclampsia: ACOG Practice Bulletin, Number 222." *Obstetrics & Gynecology* 135, no. 6 (2020): e237–e260. https://doi.org/10.1097/AOG.0000000000003891.

Osborne, Margaret. "What Is Eclampsia? Olympian Tori Bowie May Have Died from the Rare Pregnancy Condition." *Smithsonian Magazine*, June 16, 2023. https://www.smithsonianmag.com/smart-news/what-is-eclampsia-olympian-tori-bowie-may-have-died-from-the-rare-pregnancy-condition-180982388/.

Phadnis, S. V., and L. M. Irvine. "*Hydatoxi lualba*: The Worm That Wasn't!" *Journal of Obstetrics and Gynaecology* 33, no. 7 (2013): 669–670. https://doi.org/10.3109/01443615.2013.807785.

CHAPTER 12

Cohen, Elizabeth, Justin Lape, and Danielle Herman. "'Heartbreaking' Stories Go Untold, Doctors Say, as Employers 'Muzzle' Them in Wake of Abortion Ruling." CNN Health, October 12, 2022. https://www.cnn.com/2022/10/12/health/abortion-doctors-talking.

Hendrickson, John. *Life on Delay: Making Peace with a Stutter*. Penguin Random House, 2023.

Perez, Hector R., Camilo Doig-Acuña, and Joanna L. Starrels. "'Not Unless It's a Life or Death Thing': A Qualitative Study of the Health Care Experiences of Adults Who Stutter." *Journal of General Internal Medicine* 30 (2015): 1639–1644. https://doi.org/10.1007/s11606-015-3302-x.

CHAPTER 13

"ACOG Committee Opinion No. 390: Ethical Decision Making in Obstetrics and Gynecology." *Obstetrics & Gynecology* 110, no. 6 (2007): 1479–1487. https://doi.org/10.1097/01.AOG.0000291573.09193.36.

Kiang, Mathew V., Lindsey E. Carlasare, Sonoo Thadaney Israni, John J. Norcini, Junaid A. B. Zaman, and Kirsten Bibbins-Domingo. "Excess Mortality Among US Physicians During the

COVID-19 Pandemic." *JAMA Internal Medicine* 183, no. 4 (2023): 374–376. https://doi.org/10.1001/jamainternmed.2022.6308.

Scheinman, Steven J., Patrick Fleming, and Kellyann Niotis. "Oath Taking at U.S. and Canadian Medical School Ceremonies: Historical Perspectives, Current Practices, and Future Considerations." *Academic Medicine* 93, no. 9 (2018): 1301–1306. https://doi.org/10.1097/ACM.0000000000002097.

CHAPTER 14

Goodman, J. David. "Abortion Ruling Keeps Texas Doctors Afraid of Prosecution." *New York Times*, December 13, 2023. https://www.nytimes.com/2023/12/13/us/texas-abortion-doctor-prosecution.html.

"Prediction and Prevention of Spontaneous Preterm Birth: ACOG Practice Bulletin, Number 234." *Obstetrics & Gynecology* 138, no. 2 (2021): e65–e90. https://doi.org/10.1097/AOG.0000000000004479.

Sepper, Elizabeth, Kari White, and Anitra Beasley. "The Texas Medical Board and the Futility of Medical Exceptions to Abortion Bans." *JAMA* 331, no. 24 (2024): 2073–2074. https://doi.org/10.1001/jama.2024.9027.

CHAPTER 15

Sonenberg, Andrea, and Diana J. Mason. "Maternity Care Deserts in the US." *JAMA Health Forum* 4, no. 1 (2023): e225541. https://doi.org/10.1001/jamahealthforum.2022.5541.

Stolberg, Sheryl Gay. "As Abortion Laws Drive Obstetricians from Red States, Maternity Care Suffers." *New York Times*, September 6, 2023.

Stoneburner, Ashley, Ripley Lucas, Jazmin Fontenot, Christina Brigance, Erin Jones, and Andrea L. DeMaria. *Nowhere to Go: Maternity Care Deserts Across the US.* Report No 4. March of Dimes, 2024. https://www.marchofdimes.org/maternity-care-deserts-report.

CHAPTER 16

American College of Obstetricians and Gynecologists and Society for Maternal-Fetal Medicine. "Obstetric Care Consensus No. 6: Periviable Birth." *Obstetrics & Gynecology* 130, no. 4 (2017): e187–e199. https://doi.org/10.1097/AOG.0000000000002352.

Shah, Payal, and Akila Radhakrishnan. "It's Time to Call Abortion Bans What They Are—Torture and Cruelty." *The Nation*, June 9, 2023. https://www.thenation.com/article/society/abortion-bans-torture-cruelty/.

Younge, Noelle, Ricki F. Goldstein, Carla M. Bann, Susan R. Hintz, Ravi M. Patel, P. Brian Smith, et al. "Survival and Neurodevelopmental Outcomes Among Periviable Infants." *New England Journal of Medicine* 376, no. 7 (2017): 617–628. https://doi.org/10.1056/NEJMoa1605566.

Index